Collins ne

Yoga

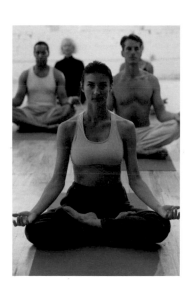

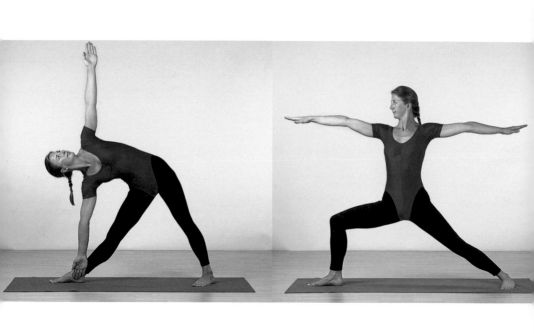

Collins need to know?

Yoga

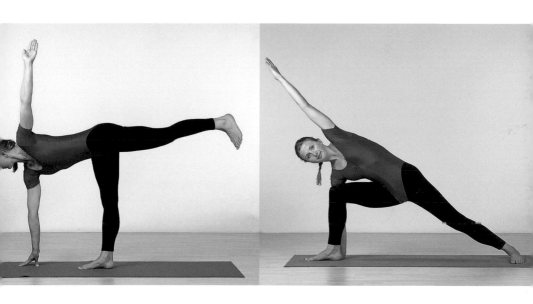

All the tips and techniques you need
to get healthy in mind and body

Patricia A. Ralston and Caroline Smart

First published in 2005 by
Collins, an imprint of
HarperCollins*Publishers*
77-85 Fulham Palace Road
Hammersmith, London W6 8JB

The Collins website address is: www.collins.co.uk

Collins is a registered trademark of HarperCollins Publishers Limited.

09 08 07 06 05
6   5   4   3   2   1

Yoga can cause bodily injury so you should consult your doctor prior to attempting any of the
exercises contained in this book. The authors and publisher do not accept liability for any injury
suffered as a result of negligence in performing the exercises contained in this book. Exercises
contained in this book are carried out at your own risk and may not be suitable for every reader.

The information contained in this book, including addresses, telephone numbers and website details,
is correct at the time of going to press but the publisher cannot accept responsibility for any
subsequent changes.

A catalogue record for this book is available from the British Library

Created by: The Printer's Devil, Glasgow
Asana photography: Richard Palmer
Other photography: BlackEye Photography, except for Getty Images (pp. 1, 4, 7, 8, 10, 11, 12, 13, 14
[top], 16, 18, 20, 21 [top], 23 [top], 24, 25, 26, 30, 156, 161, 162, 164, 174, 176, 177 [bottom], 179,
180, 182) and Artville (pp. 15, 166, 177 [top], 185)
Model: Bella Galt (asanas)
Model's clothing supplied by: Ealing Dance Centre, London
Cover design: Cook Design
Front cover photograph: Getty Images/Jack Ambrose

ISBN 0 00 719091 3

Much of the material in this book is based on Collins *Gem Yoga*, 1999

Colour reproduction by Colourscan, Singapore
Printed and bound by Printing Express Ltd, Hong Kong

contents

Introduction

Many people are wary of yoga. They either imagine it as a slightly weird Eastern religion practised by would-be hippies or else see it as a form of soft physical exercise practised by middle-aged ladies in leotards and tights.

Benefits to mind and body

Both these preconceptions mean that yoga is sometimes ridiculed or dismissed out of hand. But once discovered for what it is – an extremely effective and beneficial form of exercise, both for the body and mind – the student will incorporate yoga almost unconsciously into his or her way of life and reap the benefits that come from doing so.

Yoga brings not only an awareness to your body – how you sit, how you stand, how you breathe – but it also focuses your attention on your mind, letting you learn how to relax and how to recognise and still a racing mind filled with the problems of the day.

Yoga without preconceptions

If you can, try to approach yoga without any preconceptions. You can take from it as much or as little as you want. If you just want something to make you more supple, to stop that scrunched-up feeling in your neck after a hard day's work hunched over a desk, then try attending a beginner's class and feel the gentle stretching you can get from practising the postures. You may find yourself wanting to explore other aspects of yoga: the breathing, the philosophy, the literature.

As much or as little as you want is there to be discovered. But just as your yoga teacher will tell you when referring to the postures, 'Only do what feels right for you'.

The selection of postures included in this book have been chosen to illustrate the ones that you are likely to be taught in a hatha yoga class. We have omitted some of the more difficult postures, which should be learned only under the supervision of a properly qualified yoga teacher.

Patricia A. Ralston
Caroline Smart

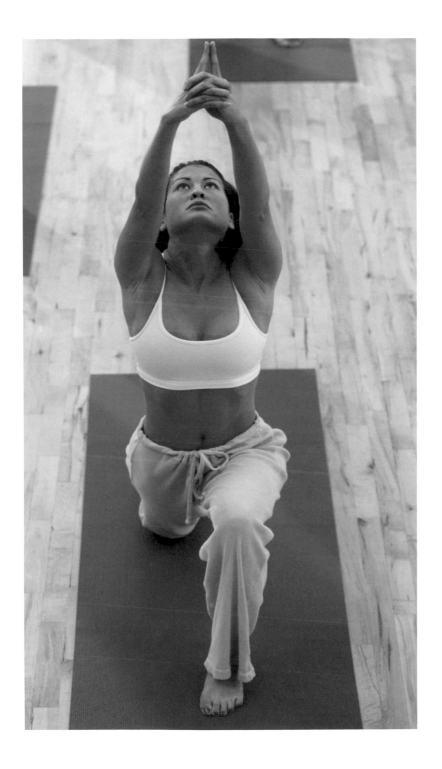

hatha

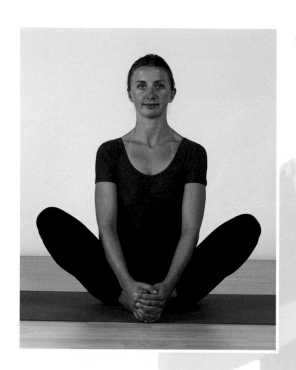

yoga

When people in the West refer to yoga, they are generally talking about hatha yoga. *Hatha* means force or will and this type of yoga is thus known as the yoga of will. The hatha yoga student aims to gain mastery over his or her body by practising the postures (*asanas*) and by breath control (*pranayama*). This chapter outlines the benefits of hatha yoga.

What is hatha yoga?

Hatha yoga is the style of yoga that is taught most often in classes in the West. It is a physical regime designed to strengthen and cleanse the body in preparation for gaining control of the mind through meditation.

Postures and breathing

The student of hatha yoga gains mastery over their body through practising the postures (*asanas*) and through breath control (*pranayama*). Once the body is under control, the student can turn their attention to gaining control over the mind by meditation. When this has been achieved, they are ready to proceed along the eightfold path and join the path of Raja yoga (see p. 185). However, most of us are content to stay with the postures and breathing to gain a better sense of wellbeing.

Yoga vs physical exercise

Physical exercise aims primarily to tone the body, building strength, stamina and flexibility through exercise; the mind does not have to be engaged. Purely physical exercises can be done almost without thinking, even while listening to

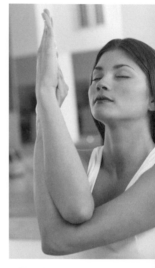

▲ Yoga blends the physical, the mental and the spiritual and the emphasis you want to place on each element is up to you.

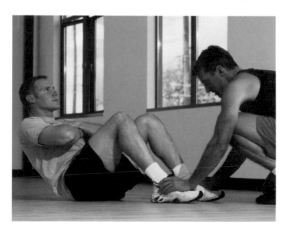

◄ Working out in the gym emphasizes the physical over the mental with its concentration on 'reps' – the repetition of the same movement until exhaustion.

▶ Physical exercises often target one specific area without being applied to the body as a whole. Also muscle bulk is built up without taking flexibility into consideration.

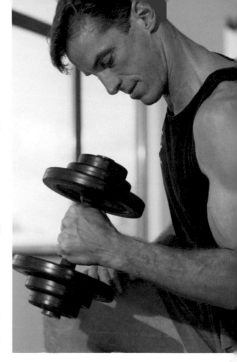

music or watching TV. And there is not always a sense of balance: for instance, a backbend might not be counterbalanced by a forward bend, resulting in a potential distortion in the body.

Yoga encompasses both body and mind. Although the asanas are physical postures, they must be approached with concentration and awareness. They are not just a means to physical fitness: they also lead to a well-balanced, flexible body and a clear mind. Breath control is also important.

In all, the harnessing of the body makes possible the harnessing of the mind so letting the student go on to pursue the spiritual side of yoga if they choose.

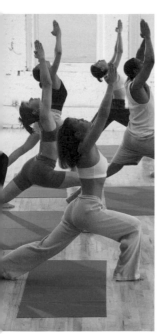

▲ Yoga is not competitive. It is about discovering your own body and yourself.

Approaching the postures

Each posture should be approached as though you are doing it for the first time. It should not be like doing mindlessly repetitive exercises like press-ups – both mind and body are involved.

There should be no anticipation, otherwise your movements become purely automatic and you lose awareness of what your body is doing. You should take stock of how you feel, and of how your breath comes and goes; nothing should be rushed.

Nor should you look around in class to see how anyone else is doing. You should concentrate on doing just as much of the posture as you are able, without forcing.

Who can do yoga?

One of the great things about yoga is that anyone can take it up and benefit from it. You might be very stiff and wonder how you will ever manage a seated forward bend. The answer is

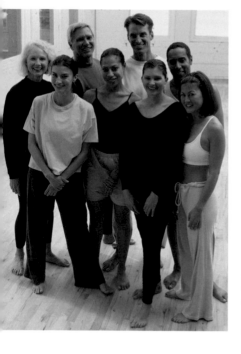

you must only do as much as your body allows. In quite a short time and with regular practice you will find yourself becoming more supple and things you found impossible in your first class come more and more within your grasp.

Yoga is not about comparing yourself to others in the class – even if they look as though they can bend in two!

What benefits are there?

The benefits of hatha yoga, working on both body and mind, cannot be underestimated. Compare a depressed person, often weighed

◀ Regardless of your age, sex or experience when starting, over time and with regular practice, yoga will bring you both mental and physical benefits.

MUST KNOW

Yoga is ideal for everyone!
● **Children:** although youngsters are naturally supple, postures can help them build concentration.
● **Stress sufferers:** breathing and relaxation techniques are beneficial in coping with stress.
● **Pregnant women:** yoga can help prepare for birth – postures are adaptable for most stages and breathing techniques can help in labour.
● **The disabled:** many postures can be adapted to suit special needs without losing any of the benefits.
● **The overweight:** regular, gentle practice increases your feeling of wellbeing and encourages a more balanced approach to life and food. Many of the postures work on regulating the thyroid gland which dictates how your body uses up food.
● **Seniors:** the gentle approach to the postures lends itself to those of more advanced years and regular practice improves all-over flexibility.

down by worry, with shoulders and neck tensed and hunched. They may find it difficult to concentrate or make decisions. They have no energy and tend to neglect their bodies.

However, a happy person walks with shoulders relaxed and wide, their spine straight. Their minds are focused on what they are doing and they have no problems making decisions. Yoga promotes this feeling of wellbeing by toning both the body and the mind.

However, the postures do not just work to tone and reshape the outside of the body – they also stimulate all of the internal organs and even revitalize the nervous system.

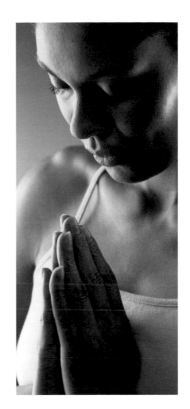

▶ Mentally, yoga calms and disciplines the mind, improves concentration and counteracts stress, helps you control your emotions and promotes a positive happy attitude.

BENEFITS

- Creates energy and improves stamina, fitness and concentration.
- Increases awareness of your body.
- Keeps the body flexible so energy flows freely.
- Works on internal organs and the endocrine system, and regulates metabolism.
- Improves digestive and elimination processes.
- Rejuvenates, decreases tension and teaches relaxation.
- Improves posture and delays the ageing process.
- Helps reduce excess fat.
- Improves circulation and skin tone.
- Needs no expensive equipment to practise.
- Postures provide a full, balanced range of motion.

The spine

You are as old as your spine is flexible, and in yoga particular attention is paid to the spine. The spine houses the spinal cord which carries instructions from the brain to the rest of the body and it is important to keep it in good working order. Many asanas work on the spine by bending it forward, backward and through twisting movements. The spinal-flexing exercises ensure the nerves get a good blood supply and there is none of the tension which often leads to back problems. Any vertebral irregularity is realigned by the twisting postures.

The endocrine system

This system controls the glands and hormones in the body. A healthy endocrine system is vital as it can affect our appearance, disposition and behaviour. Growth, body shape and the way in which the body uses food are also influenced by the endocrine system.

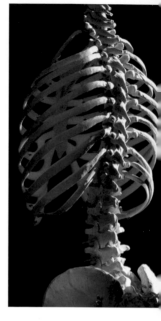

▲ The gentle curves of the normal adult spine protect it from jarring.

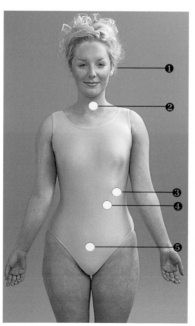

◄ The glands of the endocrine system:

❶ The pituitary gland (at the base of the brain) regulates the growth of the entire body and the development and functioning of the sex glands.

❷ The thyroid gland controls body growth and metabolism – the rate at which the body uses food and oxygen.

❸ The adrenal glands produces adrenalin. This hormone is released in conditions of stress and causes increased heartbeat, breathing, etc.

❹ The pancreas controls body growth and metabolism – the rate at which the body uses food and oxygen.

❺ The sex glands (ovaries in females, testes in males) are vital in developing gender characteristics.

Specific postures work on different glands, mainly by increasing the blood supply to them. This increased blood supply brings with it oxygen and nutrients vital for ensuring the glands' healthy working. A well-balanced yoga routine should ensure the smooth running of all these glands. For example, inverted (upside down) poses bring blood to the brain and stimulate the pituitary gland; they also cause the chin to press into the neck, stimulating and regulating the thyroid gland most effectively.

The importance of breathing

Breathing is vital in yoga. Control of the breath leads to control of the mind and it is this which distinguishes yoga from purely physical exercise.

Most of us only use perhaps a third of our lung capacity, at the top of the lungs, so we take in very little air which is so essential to the health of the body and internal organs.

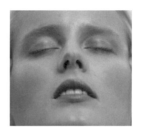

▲ Learning how to breathe correctly – and fully – is a vital part of learning how to do each asana correctly.

Breathing should involve the upper lungs (beneath the collarbones), the middle part where the ribcage expands, and the bottom section. Breathing into this bottom section is known as abdominal breathing, and brings the maximum amount of air to the largest area of the lungs. This breathing is slow and deep.

Breathing should be done only through the nose. Nostril hairs filter dust particles and the mucous lining helps kill germs. As air travels up the nasal passages it is warmed, ready to be taken into the lungs. If you breathe through your mouth all these benefits are lost.

MUST KNOW

Breathing and postures

Awareness of breathing is important while undertaking the postures. Both the inhalation (breathing in) and exhalation (breathing out) are used to help the body into each pose. Paying special attention to and being aware of your breathing rhythm lets you feel how it helps.

want to know **more?**

Take it to the next level...

Go to...
▶ **The yoga class** – page 18
▶ **Types of yoga** – pages 21 and 183
▶ **Breathing exercises** – page 166

Other sources
▶ **Qualified yoga teacher**
   to answer basic queries about hatha yoga
▶ **Videos/DVDs**
   on hatha yoga
▶ **Magazines**
   for specialist features
▶ **Internet**
   for details of different yoga styles
▶ **Publications**
   visit www.thorsons.com for books on yoga

learning

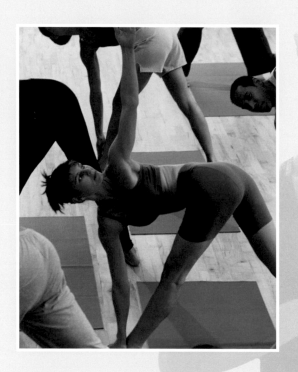

yoga

You may decide to teach yourself yoga at home, perhaps using one of the many books or videos that are now available. This is certainly a good way to find out about yoga, but you shouldn't underestimate the benefits of attending a class. In this chapter, we'll look at choosing a suitable class and what to expect from it.

The yoga class

Whether you are new to yoga or an experienced practitioner, attending a class under the guidance of a qualified teacher brings a wide range of benefits that allow you to put more into your practice while also getting more out of it.

The benefits

For beginners, the most obvious benefit of attending a yoga class is that the teacher is there to teach you the postures, and then make sure that you perform them correctly.

A good teacher can spot imbalances – feet too close together or too far apart, or your bottom sticking out and throwing out the whole balance and benefit of the posture. A teacher talking you through a posture will bring out its subtle aspects and make you aware of which parts of your body are being stretched and which should be relaxed. They will also talk you through the breathing.

It is difficult to be aware of all this practising on your own. And the benefits of encouragement in a class are very real. But it is important to find a style and a class that suits you. It may take some time, but it is worth looking around to see what is available in your area.

▼ If new to yoga, you should consider learning the basics under the guidance of an experienced teacher. Once you feel comfortable with the postures and breathing rhythms taught in your class, then you'll be able to practice more successfully on your own.

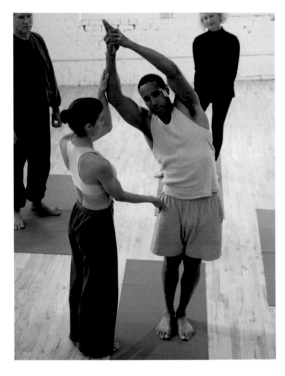

LEARNING YOGA

18

A good teacher...

- gives a varied and balanced class.
- judges the mood of the class and adjusts the class plan to suit it.
- develops the postures over a number of weeks.
- keeps the students motivated.
- can explain the postures and make you aware of what you should feel when you do each one.
- can explain clearly how the posture works on the body and describe the benefits.
- observes students and rectifies faults in a positive, non-critical way. If they need to touch the student, this is done very gently with very little actual pressure.
- warns who ought not to try a posture, e.g. high-blood-pressure sufferers, those menstruating.
- can modify postures for students with specific problems or conditions, e.g. neck, back, physical disability, arthritis or pregnancy.

Finding a class

You can find out about yoga classes in your area from a number of readily available sources.

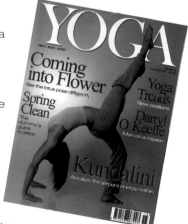

Yoga associations

The British Wheel of Yoga lists local classes while the Scottish Yoga Teachers' Association gives lists of hatha yoga classes in Scotland. Contact details of these bodies are in the **Need to know more?** section on pages 188–89.

Magazines

Yoga magazine, published monthly in the UK, lists classes. Its classified ads section also features a variety of classes and courses in the UK, as well as yoga holidays abroad.

Local authorities and leisure centres

Many local authorities and leisure centres offer classes. Leisure centres often have mats so you

▲ Magazines such as *Yoga* are a useful source of classes in your area, as are the notice boards of your local health and leisure centres. Regardless of your age, experience or sex, you should be able to find a class that suits you.

don't have to take one. In some private classes, you pay for a session which can last around four or six weeks.

Other information sources

Health-food shops, alternative bookshops and local shops often have notice boards with details of classes, as do many local libraries.

Practical considerations

When deciding which yoga class is best for you, there are a number of points you should think about.

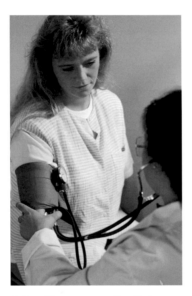

▲ As with any new pastime that can be physically demanding, it's worth consulting your doctor before starting your yoga class if you haven't been active in the past or if you have an existing medical condition.

Is there a convenient class nearby?

Is it easy to get to, or would you have to depend on public transport? Going out on a cold winter's night can be very unappealing! Lunchtime classes may sound ideal but will you have to rush from work, get changed then rush back? An evening class may start too early to let you get home, eat and go out again. You should always leave at least an hour and a half after eating a light meal. And would an evening class finish so late that you would almost be asleep by the end?

How long is the class?

Ideally, a class should last about ninety minutes. An hour is quite short and more importantly, there may not be enough time for a proper relaxation session at the end.

WATCH OUT!

Check the venue

It is always worth going to see where the class is actually held. It might be in a cold, draughty church hall. On the other hand, a leisure centre might be quite noisy with other classes going on around you.

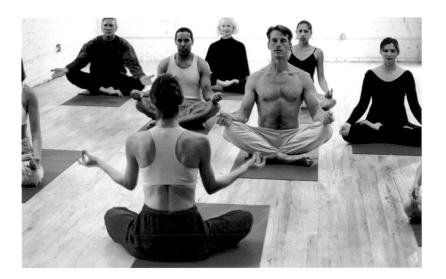

Types of yoga teaching

A further important consideration is whether the actual style of yoga being taught the right one for you. As we discussed in the previous chapter, most classes in the West teach Hatha yoga but not all are the same.

Yoga is a blend of the physical, the mental and the spiritual and many teachers develop a particular slant, emphasising one aspect over another. Ideally, you will find a teacher who offers a balanced class that you feel comfortable in.

Moreover, in addition to Hatha yoga, there are five other yoga styles you may come across and it is worth exploring each to see which you think would be most suitable for you.

Iyengar yoga

Based on the teachings of B. K. S. Iyengar, this style of yoga is vigorous and includes the use of a variety of props – blocks (both foam and wooden), chairs and belts. A great deal of attention is paid to the details of the postures and students progress from beginners to advanced. Students are taught to jump into the

▲ Although all work with the same basic postures, yoga teachers often adapt them to suit their individual approaches and personal styles.

▼ Millions of students across the globe have followed the teachings of B. K. S. Iyengar and there are Iyengar institutes and centres in the UK, across Europe, in North America, the Antipodes as well as in India. *Light on Yoga* is his classic text.

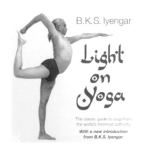

standing poses. Iyengar teachers undergo an specialized teacher-training course to qualify.

Kundalini yoga

This aims to bring forth the energy, kundalini, stored at the base of the spine. It travels up the spine to the crown of the head. The postures and breathing techniques clear the way for this energy to travel. Chanting and meditation also play a part in arousing the energy.

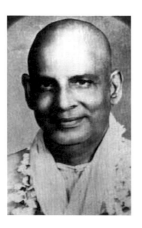

▲ Swami Sivananda, who is considered one of the greatest and most prolific yoga masters of the 20th century and the inspiration behind Sivananda yoga.

Sivananda yoga

Founded by Swami Sivananda, this style combines all the paths of yoga: asana, pranayama, selfless service, prayer, chanting, meditation and self-study.

Ashtanga yoga or power yoga

This type of yoga calls for strength, flexibility and stamina. Postures are done in a series linked by the breath. Ashtanga yoga aims to strengthen and purify the nervous system, allowing energy, *prana*, to flow up through the spine.

Viniyoga

Developed by T. K. V. Desikachar, this style works with breath, movement, sound, ritual and meditation. Attention is focused on the spine and postures are tailored to suit the needs of each student. Teaching is person-centred and taught on a one-to-one basis.

For details of teachers in your area, see **Need to know more?** on pages 188–89.

MUST KNOW

The Internet

The Internet is a great way to find out more about the different schools of yoga and their teachings. Many sites cover the different aspects of each style, with examples of the postures and step-by-step instructions.

Outfits and equipment

For beginners, one of the best things about yoga is that you don't need to invest heavily in specialized kit to get started.

Clothing

You should wear comfortable clothing – leggings and a tee-shirt, leotard or loose cotton trousers. You don't need any kind of footwear: your bare feet will give a good grip on the floor and maximum awareness coming through the soles of your feet. Take a jumper or fleece and a pair of socks to wear during the relaxation session when your body cools down very quickly.

Equipment

A non-slip mat is also very useful, letting you do the standing postures without slipping, and providing a firm base for the standing and balance postures. The teacher will be able to tell you where you can buy one and may be able to order it for you.

You should also take a blanket (a plaid is ideal). It can be used for the seated and lying-down postures. It can also be folded and used for seated postures where you need to prop your hip up on one side. It also keeps you warm during the closing relaxation period.

Some teachers use foam blocks. These are useful to put under your buttocks when you are sitting with crossed legs and your knees should ideally be touching the ground. Blocks can also be used to support yourself when you need to put your hand on the ground but cannot quite stretch down far enough.

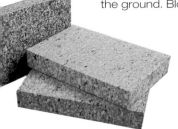

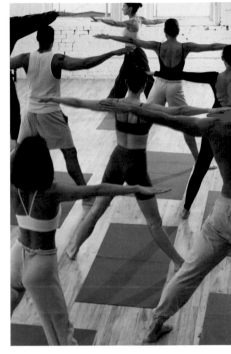

▲ Apart from a mat, you need little to get started with yoga other than comfortable clothing.

WATCH OUT!

What not to wear
Don't wear anything too baggy – the teacher needs to be able to see what your arms and legs are doing to check that you are performing the posture correctly. Also, don't wear your watch or loose jewellery as it can be distracting.

What to expect in class

Classes tend to be predominantly female for hatha yoga, with more men attending Iyengar and Ashtanga (Power) yoga classes. However, this should not put anyone off from attending the type of class they prefer. The size of a class can vary from five to about thirty people. There must be enough room for people to lie down and be able to stretch their arms out to the side. The teacher will explain each posture and demonstrate it before allowing the class to attempt it. The teacher will then talk the class through the posture, observing each of the students to make sure they are doing it correctly.

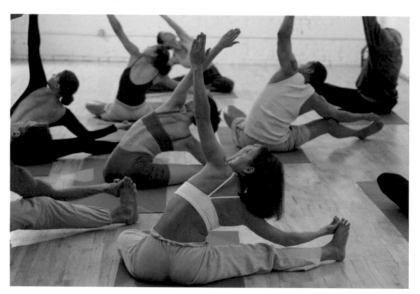

BENEFITS

- It gets you fit and toned, and helps you build up your strength.
- It helps you to regulate weight.
- It helps you to become more supple.
- It can alleviate or reduce back problems.
- You will learn how to relax effectively.
- It helps relieve stress.
- It is a form of exercise that is gentle but effective.
- It lets you try something different.

▲ Yoga classes often have a preponderance of women despite the fact that both sexes benefit greatly from the practice. The absence – or presence – of men should not inhibit you from joining the class you want.

▶ Hatha yoga may look a very slow activity but the postures require strength and it can benefit men, who are often strong but lack suppleness.

Class routine

A well-structured class generally consists of:

● A warming-up session: perhaps including the cleansing and complete breaths.

● A series of balanced postures: promoting stamina, strength, balance, suppleness, and a quiet mind.

● A mix of postures: standing, seated, balancing, backbends, twists, inverted postures.

● Relaxation.

Yoga offers so much that it is worth putting in as much effort as possible. If you do, you will soon be reaping the benefits: attending a yoga class should leave you feeling balanced and better physically, mentally and emotionally.

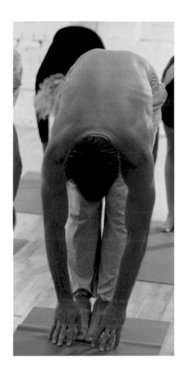

MUST KNOW

A good student...

● tries to attend classes regularly.

● listens to the teacher.

● comes to each posture as though for the first time and is aware of how each part of their body is reacting.

● only goes as far as their body allows.

● pays attention to their breath, using it to surrender into the pose.

● concentrates fully on doing the postures, putting aside any worries and problems.

● practises the postures at home.

● is open to new ideas that the teacher offers.

want to know more?

Take it to the next level...

Go to...

▶ **Physical benefits of yoga** – page 12

▶ **Asana basics** – page 28

▶ **Home session** – page 176

Other sources

▶ **Videos/DVDs**
   to supplement your class teaching

▶ **Local library/sports centre**
   for local classes

▶ **Magazines**
   for lists of local teachers

▶ **Internet**
   for equipment suppliers

▶ **Publications**
   visit www.thorsons.com for books on yoga

about

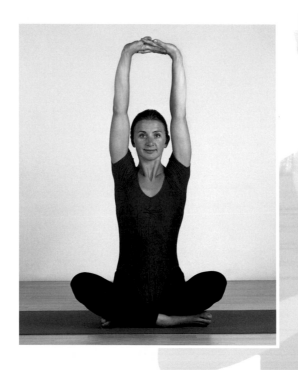

asanas

Yoga postures are known as *asanas* in Sanskrit. They are not just a random series of movements: each works in harmony with the others to help achieve a healthy physicial and mental state. This chapter explores the background to practising the asanas correctly, outlining the principles of balance between postures and the importance of correct breathing.

Asana basics

Modern hatha yoga teaching puts the number of asanas at around 200. But an earlier manual on the subject says there are 32 postures that are useful to human beings – a much more manageable number for the average yoga student!

Asana names

When you practise yoga you will hear the postures' Sanskrit names used as well as their translations. It is useful to know both as many teachers, especially of the Iyengar method (see p. 21), frequently refer to the Sanskrit names, as do many yoga books.

MUST KNOW

'Steady pose'

Asana means 'steady pose'. The postures, once mastered, are to be held steady for some time.

Some people find the asanas' Sanskrit names confusing and intimidating. But while they may seem daunting at first, they don't take long to memorize. We have listed both English and Sanskrit asana names in a glossary at the back of the book (see pp. 186–87). To ease yourself over any difficulty, it is worth remembering that the names of the postures usually refer to an animal (such as cobra, cat, locust) or a shape (for example, triangle or half moon).

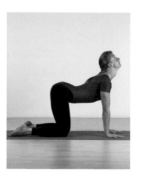 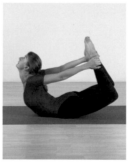

◀ Keep the Sanskrit meaning in mind when doing each asana so you have an overall image of what the posture should look like: far left, the Arched Cat and left, the Bow.

Re-educating your body

Although yoga is ancient, it offers lessons on how to cope with life in a fast age when we seem to be losing touch with our bodies. Nowadays both children and adults spend many hours a day sitting at desks, often in front of computer screens. The longer we do this, the more we slouch, neck forward, shoulders rounded, letting the muscles of the spine slacken. Tension builds up in all these areas.

If you watch a six-month-old baby learning to sit, you can see how easily and naturally it sits up with a beautifully straight spine. But if you try to imitate this by sitting on the floor, do you find your back becoming tired? You might feel some muscular discomfort and just long to let your spine collapse into its usual slump.

The same may be true of how you stand. Good posture is something we lose over the years as age, gravity and habit take a hold. Yoga postures go back to these very basic aspects and re-educate the body, making it aware of how it should really be feeling.

Once you have learnt these basics, you will find it hard to ignore bad habits in the future. Even if you do give in to them, you will still be aware of them!

▲ The basic standing posture, Tadasana (Mountain), teaches you how to stand correctly.

Asanas in balance

As has been mentioned before, yoga postures are not done individually. Balance is the key to yoga. Postures are done so that they put the body through the whole range of movements.

In class, a bend to the right will always be counterbalanced by a bend to the left; a backbend will be followed by a forward bend; and a twist to the left will be followed by a twist to the right.

A good teacher always presents a well-balanced class where the selection of postures leaves you refreshed and revitalized, not exhausted and drained of energy.

A balanced session should therefore include a mixture of standing, lying, inverted, backbends, seated and balancing postures, and bear in mind some of the basic guidelines outlined overleaf.

WATCH OUT!

Don't stand for it
Don't include too many standing postures in a session. They promote strength and may encourage aggression. You should never push yourself too far, even trying to compete with what you have achieved before.

MUST KNOW

Basic guidelines for a balanced session

- Always begin with a warming-up session to limber up and loosen the spine and joints.
- Hold each posture for a few seconds. Rest for a moment or two between postures and move slowly and gracefully.
- Balance forward bends with backward bends.
- If you compress one part of the body in a posture, then you must extend it in a counterpose.
- Always practise to each side in postures such as Triangle (Trikonasana) or the twists.
- Leave strong backbends such as Cobra (Bhujangasana) or Locust (Salabhasana) until quite well into the session. Your spine and hips need time to loosen and limber up before tackling these.
- End a session with a quietening, closing down pose such as Seated Forward Bend (Paschimottanasana). Allow a few minutes' relaxation at the end of the session.

Breathing

When we talk of breathing here, we are not referring to *pranayama* or other yogic breathing techniques; these are discussed separately in the chapter on Yogic Breath on p. 162. Breathing in the context of asanas is to raise energy and relax into the posture.

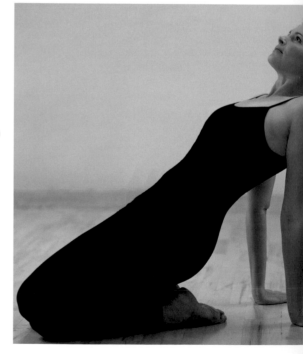

▶The in-breath is used to move the body into the posture; exhalation, which removes impurities from the body, is used to relax into the posture.

What makes yoga unique as an exercise system is that the breath plays a major part in how each posture is approached. The breath is used to explore and develop the postures.

Breathing consists of the in-breath (inhalation) and the out-breath (exhalation).

Inhalation

Inhalation, which brings vital oxygen into the body, is energizing. In-breath expands, lengthens and helps upward movement. For example, you would raise arms on an in-breath but lower them on an out-breath. You would use the in-breath to lift out of a seated forward bend.

Exhalation

Out-breath releases tension, and helps downward movement. For example, you would breathe out going into a seated forward bend. Once you were in the pose you would use another out-breath to relax further into the forward bend.

WATCH OUT!

Don't forget
Because breathing plays such an important part in yoga, it is important not to neglect it. This is especially important when learning at home from a book or video. Pay attention to the breathing instructions for each posture – you will find that they help.

MUST KNOW

Nasal breathing
While performing the postures breathing should be done through the nose, unless otherwise advised.

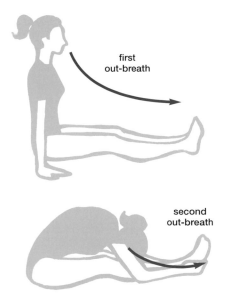

first
out-breath

second
out-breath

◀ Understanding how the correct type of breath helps you complete each posture is vital to successful yoga. The seated forward bend, for example, uses the out-breath both to move into the posture and then to relax further into it.

Eye exercises

Exercise 1

Sit in a comfortable pose with your spine straight, shoulders relaxed and back, chin parallel to the floor and eyes looking straight ahead. Without moving the head, look diagonally up to the right as far as you can. Then look diagonally down to the left as far as you can. Repeat three times. Then do it in the opposite direction. Repeat three times.

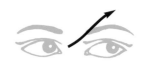

Exercise 2

Without moving the head, look straight up towards the ceiling and then down to the floor. Repeat three times.

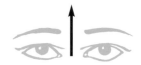

Exercise 3

Without moving the head, look as far to the right as you can, then look as far to the left as you can. Repeat three times.

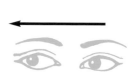

Exercise 4

Move the eyes in a clockwise circular motion. You want to make the biggest circle as possible with your eyes. Repeat three times. Then circle anti-clockwise. Repeat three times.

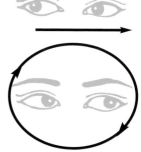

Exercise 5

Stretch your left arm out in front of you at eye level, with the index finger pointing up. Place your right index finger half way between the left finger and your eyes. Focus both eyes first of the farther left index finger, then focus both eyes on the closer right index finger. Repeat three times.

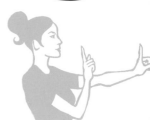

WATCH OUT!

Eye exercises
These exercises should not be done while wearing contact lenses.

Neck exercises

Exercise 1

Sit in a comfortable pose with your spine straight, shoulders relaxed and back, chin parallel to the floor, eyes looking straight ahead. Without moving your shoulders, turn your head as far as you can to the right, trying to look at the wall behind you. Then turn your head as far as you can to the left, making sure that the shoulders do not move. Repeat four times in each direction.

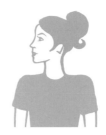

Exercise 2

Keeping your shoulders still, drop your head forward to your chest, then take it up and back so that you are looking at the ceiling. Try not to scrunch the back of the neck, imagine you have a rolled-up towel wedged there. Repeat both movements four times.

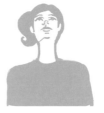

Exercise 3

With eyes looking straight ahead, drop your head sideways as though your right ear is trying to touch your right shoulder. Don't be tempted to lift the shoulder to meet the ear! Then repeat on the left side. Repeat four times on each side.

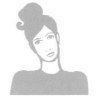

Exercise 4

Let your head drop forward to your chest. Then roll head round to the right in a wide circular movement. Perform four entire circles to the right then repeat the same circular movement to the left. Take care not to move the shoulders.

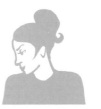

WATCH OUT!

Neck exercises
Take care if you have osteoporosis, osteoarthritis, arthritis or ear problems.

the

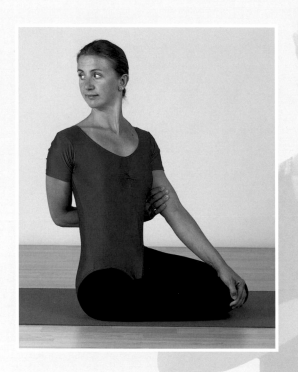

asanas

Asanas are at the core of hatha yoga. Each has been carefully studied and developed to help promote a healthy body and balanced mind. On the following pages you will find a broad range of asanas grouped according to the basic posture style (twists, backbends, balances, etc.). Each style varies in complexity from the basic through to the challenging.

▶ Kummerasana *Cat*

This is a nice gentle way to get the whole of the spine moving and to coordinate both breath and movement. All the movement is along the length of the spine – arms stay straight and still. It is particularly good for toning up the female reproductive organs. Focus on spreading your bottom as you breathe in and raise your head.

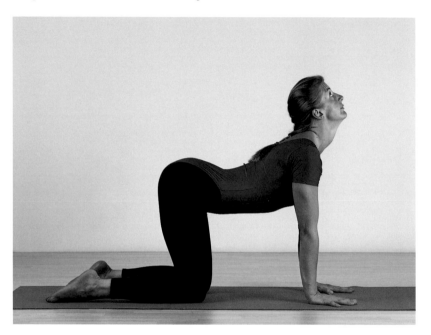

BENEFITS

- Brings flexibility to the spine.
- Strengthens the back and arms.
- Tones and firms buttock and hamstring muscles.
- Stimulates the nervous system.
- Improves the digestive system and the circulation.
- Helps relieve period pain.

WATCH OUT!

- Approach this posture with care if you suffer from back problems.
- Take extra care if you already have wrist or knee problems.

▶ Step 1

Start in a kneeling position, then come up onto your hands and knees.

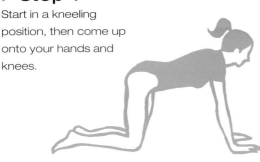

◀ Step 2

Place your hands, with palms down, on the floor directly below your shoulders. Keep them shoulder-width apart with the arms straight and the fingers pointing forward.

▲ Step 3

Position your knees so they are directly below your hips. Keep them hip-width apart, with the tops of your feet resting on the floor.

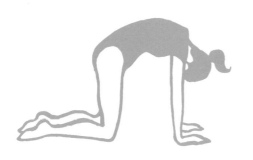

◀ Step 4

Breathe out; arch your back like an angry cat, pulling the abdominal muscles inward and upward; tuck your chin in towards your chest.

▶ Step 5

Breathe in; drop the tummy and abdominal muscles, concaving your lower back. Raise your head and look up, keeping arms straight and shoulders low. Be aware of your buttocks spreading.

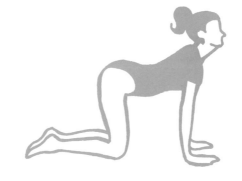

Step 6

Repeat the sequence a few times in a flowing movement, always using the breath.

► Pelvic lift

This is a good exercise for strengthening and limbering up the lower back. It is especially good if you suffer from lower back pain. It also makes you more aware of your pelvis and how its position plays a very important part in good posture both in standing and sitting. Take care not to tense the toes or jaw muscles.

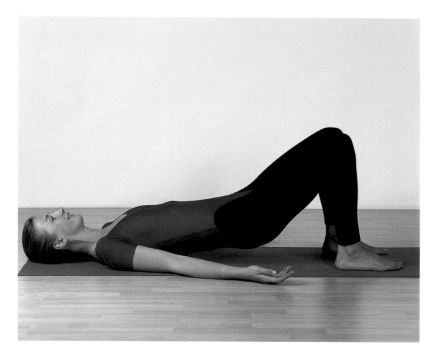

BENEFITS

- Tones the thighs, hips and buttocks.
- Strengthens the legs and the lower back.
- Tones and firms the buttock and hamstring muscles.
- Stimulates and tones the abdominal organs.
- Opens the front of the body.

WATCH OUT!

- Take care if you have an abdominal complaint.
- Approach this posture with care if you suffer from back or knee problems.

▶ Step 1

Lie with your back flat on the floor and your body in a straight line. Relax your arms by your sides, in line with your shoulders.

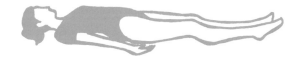

◀ Step 2

Bend your knees and put the soles of your feet flat on floor. Bring your heels close in towards your buttocks, keeping your feet hip-width apart. Your toes should be pointing forward with knees pointing up and palms facing the ceiling.

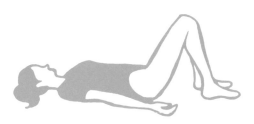

Step 3

Breathe in; raise your buttocks 15 cm (around 6 in) off the floor, tighten your thigh and buttock muscles and push the pelvis up towards the ceiling, keeping the knees pointing upwards. Feel your lower back raise up off the floor. Your chin will be tucked in.

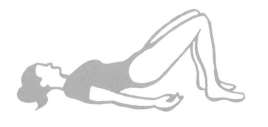

◀ Step 4

Breathe out; push your hands into the floor and, with the back of your head on the floor, slowly uncurl your spine from top to bottom onto the floor.

Step 5

Repeat several times, raising up on the in-breath and lowering on the out-breath.

▶ Butterfly

In this posture, movement should flow smoothly. The legs represent the wings of a butterfly, fluttering up and down. The front of the body should stay open throughout and the spine should stay straight, extending upwards.

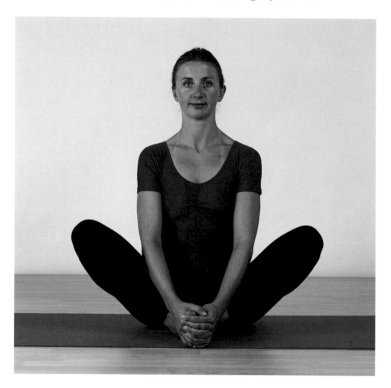

BENEFITS

- Strengthens and stimulates the leg muscles.
- Tones and tightens the thigh muscles.
- Helpful for those with sciatic problems and with lower-back pain.
- Stimulates and helps increase efficiency of the abdominal organs.

WATCH OUT!

- Take care if you have knee or hip problems.
- Do not push the knees down onto the floor as this stresses the joints.

▶ Step 1

Sit in Dandasana (as described on page 78). This position is the basis of many seated poses.

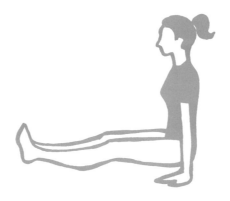

◀ Step 2

Bend the knees out to the sides, bringing the soles of the feet together in front of the body.

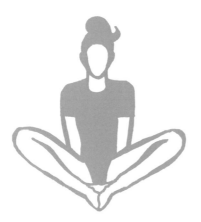

▶ Step 3

Clasp the hands together, interlinking the fingers around the toes of both feet, and draw the heels close in towards the crotch. Keep the outside edges of the feet and the little toes in contact with the floor.

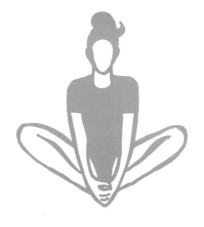

(continued)

▶ Step 4

Breathe in; stretch the
spine upwards from
the tailbone to the top
of the head; open and
expand the body.

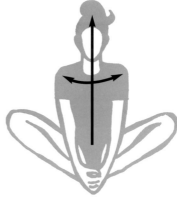

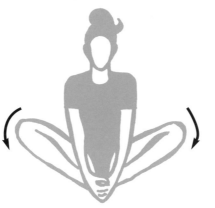

◀ Step 5

Breathe out; push the
knees out and down,
opening and
stretching the inner
muscles of the legs.
Aim to bring the
outside of the legs and
knees onto the floor.

Step 6

Repeat a few times, using the breath, as follows.
Breathe out; extend and stretch the knees out
to the sides and down. Breathe in; relax the
knees and the leg muscles.

▶ Step 7

To come out of the posture: release your hands
and breathe in. Bring your legs together in front
of your body with the knees bent. Breathe out;
extend your legs out straight, in front of your
body. Relax your arms by your sides.

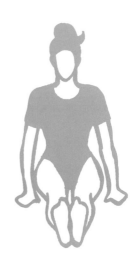

THE ASANAS

42

Surya namaskar
Salutation to the sun

This series of twelve postures is practised in a flowing sequence which combines the use of the breath.

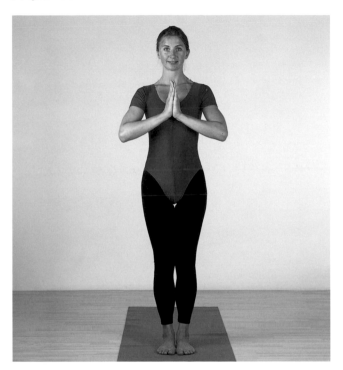

BENEFITS

- Stimulates and energizes the whole body.
- Tones and strengthens the muscles of the arms and legs.
- Increases spine flexibility and suppleness.
- Improves the circulation.
- Increases movement and joint flexibility.
- Relieves upper-body congestion.
- Tones and stimulates the internal organs.

WATCH OUT!

- Take care if you have high or low blood pressure.
- Avoid if you have severe arthritis.
- Take care if you have stiff joints or back problems.

▶ Step 1

Stand, feet together and flat on floor, body in a straight line facing forward (as in Tadasana; see page 48). Bring the hands into Namaste at mid-chest level (the prayer position; see page 73). Your fingers should point to the ceiling.

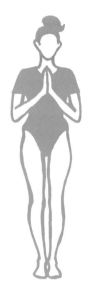

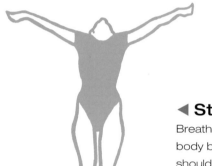

◀ Step 2

Breathe in; stretch your arms up and arch your body back from your hips, keeping your arms shoulder-width apart and palms forward. Drop your head back and look at the ceiling.

▶ Step 3

Breathe out; extend your body and arms forward, hingeing at the hips, and bring your palms down onto floor at outside of your feet; your fingers should point forward. Bring your abdomen and chest in towards your thighs, forehead to shins. Tuck your chin in towards your chest. The top of your head should be facing the floor. (This is Uttanasa; see page 69.)

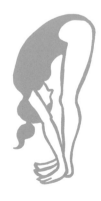

THE ASANAS

44

▶ Step 4

Breathe in; raise your
head and chest and
look forward. Stretch
your right leg back as
far as possible, then
bend your right knee
and place it on the
floor. Tuck your right
toes under; your heel

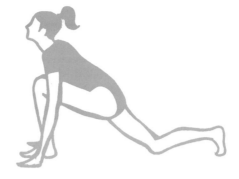

should point to the ceiling. At the same time, bend
your left knee and place it directly above your left
heel. Your left thigh should be parallel to floor, and
the sole of your left foot is flat on the floor.

▼ Step 5

Breathe out; stretch your left leg back and place
it beside your right. Push your heels down to the
floor and pull your kneecaps up. Push the backs
of your legs up to the ceiling, stretching them

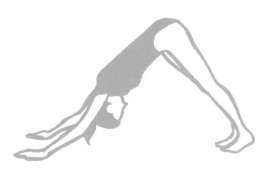

fully. At the same time
stretch your arms out
fully in front of your
body. Push your
palms and heels
down, extending your
tailbone up. Spread
your buttocks wide.
(This is Adho mukha
svanasana; see page
144.)

▶ Step 6

Push your weight onto
your palms and toes,
and lower your body:
bring your knees,
chest and chin onto
floor, keeping your
face forward.

(continued)

▶ Step 7

Breathe in; straighten
your arms and pull
your body and legs
forward, bringing your
chest through in front
of your arms. Drop
your head back and
look up to the ceiling.

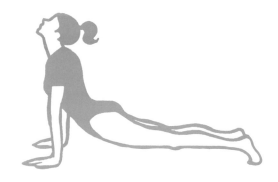

▼ Step 8

Breathe out; push your hips and tailbone up to
the ceiling. Push your thighs back, out of your
hips. Pull up your kneecaps and push your heels
down. Feel your legs
straighten and stretch.
Extend your body from
the hips down towards
the floor; the top of
your head faces the
floor. Push your tailbone
up, spreading your
buttocks. (This is Adho
mukha svanasana; see
page 144.)

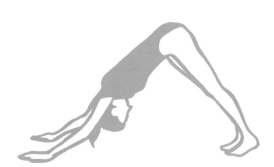

▶ Step 9

Breathe in; raise your head and
look forward, bringing your right
leg forward. Place the sole of
your foot on the floor, between
your palms, toes pointing
forward. Your right knee is now
above your right heel, with your
right thigh parallel to the floor.
Your left leg stretches out behind,
knees and toes on the floor.

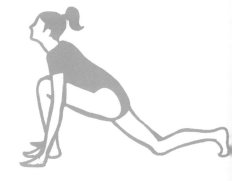

▶ Step 10

Breathe out; bring your left leg forward to place your left foot flat beside your right foot, toes forward. Straighten your legs, pull up your kneecaps and bring the front of your body in close to your legs. Place your palms down on floor beside your feet, fingers forward. (This position is Uttanasa; see page 69.)

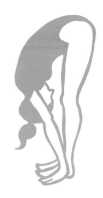

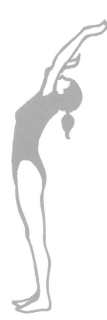

◀ Step 11

Breathe in; raise your body and arms to a vertical position, bringing your arms over your head, shoulder-width apart, with palms forward. Arch your body back at the hips, drop your head back and look up to ceiling.

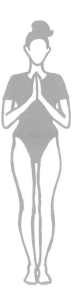

▶ Step 12

Breathe out; bring your body and arms to the vertical, lower your arms and bring your hands into Namasti at mid-chest, fingers pointing to the ceiling. Your body is now back in start position.

Step 13

Repeat the sequence to the other side, bringing the left leg back first. Then repeat the sequence a few times to each side.

▶ Tadasana *Mountain*

In Tadasana, the body is rooted to the ground and is steady like a mountain. This posture should be practised before and after all the standing postures.

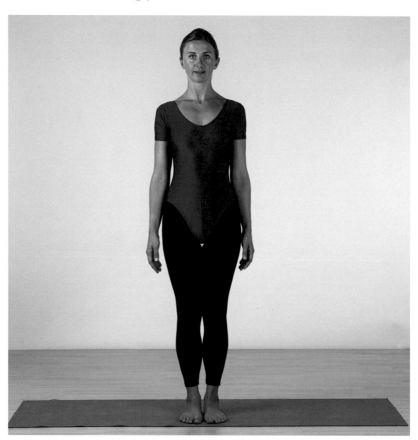

BENEFITS

- Helps balance and correct alignment in the body.
- Encourages calm within the body.
- Teaches and promotes good posture.

► Step 1

Stand with your feet together flat on the floor, with the big-toe joints and inner-ankle bones slightly touching, and your toes pointing forward. Hold your body in a straight line, facing forward. Relax your arms down by your sides, with your palms facing in towards body and fingers gently curled; your thumbnails face forward. Your body weight is distributed across the soles of both feet.

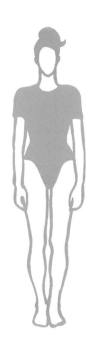

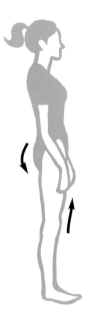

◄ Step 2

Pull your kneecaps up and lift up your leg muscles and bones. Tuck your tailbone under.

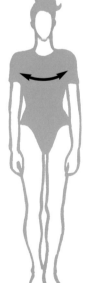

► Step 3

Lift up and open the front of your body. Relax your shoulders down and lengthen the back of your neck by lowering your chin slightly. Rest your head evenly at the top of your spine. Maintain a straight upright posture, hold and breathe normally.

▶ Vrksasana *Tree*

When practising this calming posture, concentrate on a fixed point on the floor in front of you to help you balance.

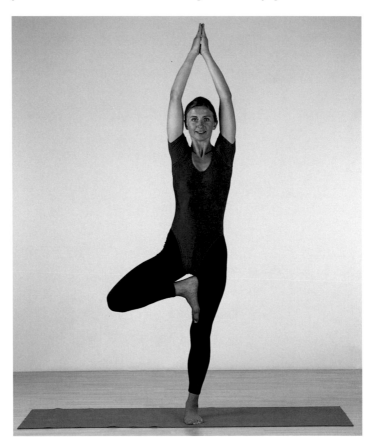

BENEFITS

- Improves general balance and coordination.
- Promotes good posture.
- Strengthens the leg muscles.
- Teaches and enhances concentration skills.

WATCH OUT!

- Do not come out of the posture quickly.
- Do not practise if you have ankle or knee problems.

THE ASANAS

50

▶ Step 1

Stand with your feet together, flat on the floor, and your body in a straight line, facing forward. Relax your arms by your sides. (See Tadasana, page 48.)

▶ Step 2

Bend your right knee up to your chest, then take your right foot and put your sole high up against your inner left thigh. Aim your right heel for the crotch, and push your heel in towards your left thigh, with right toes pointing to floor. Your right knee extends to side. Feel the stretch in your right thigh, and your hips opening out. If you suffer from vertigo, lean on a wall behind you for support.

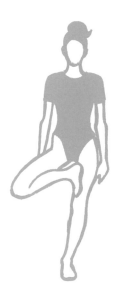

▶ Step 3

Keep your left leg straight, pulling your kneecap up. Feel your left leg strong.

(continued)

▶ Step 4

Breathe in; raise your
arms out by your
sides to shoulder level,
palms facing up.
Breathe out.

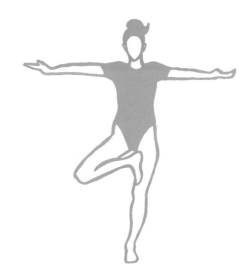

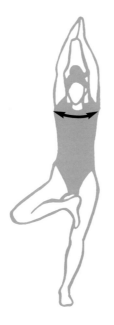

◀ Step 5

Breathe in; raise your arms, straight, above your
head and bring your palms together. Breathe
out. Stretch and extend your body upwards
from your left foot to your fingertips, lifting and
opening out at the front of the body. Hold and
breathe normally in the posture.

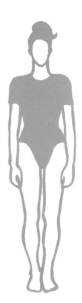

▶ Step 6

Lower your arms down by your sides, release
your right foot and replace it on the floor beside
your left.

Step 7

Repeat the posture to the other side.

Parsvakonasana
Flank stretch

This pose stretches the whole of each side of the body.
Make sure that the chest hips and legs are all in line. To do
this, focus on the upper shoulder and turn it slightly towards
the ceiling so that you open the chest. This pose keeps
ankles, knees and thighs in shape.

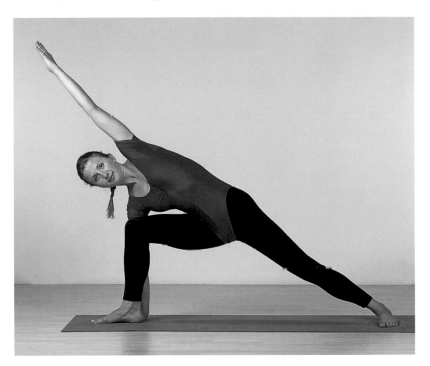

BENEFITS

- Helps with hip and lower-back problems.
- Stimulates digestion.
- Strengthens the legs and feet.
- Helpful for respiratory problems.

WATCH OUT!

- Do not strain the neck or shoulder.
- Take care if you have hip or back problems.

▶ Step 1

Stand with your feet together, flat on the floor, and your body in a straight line, facing forward. Relax your arms by your sides. (See Tadasana, page 48.)

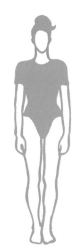

◀ Step 2

Take your feet 1.2 m (4 ft) apart. Turn your right foot out to a 90° angle and your left foot in to 45° (your right heel is in line with your left instep).

▶ Step 3

Breathe in; raise your arms out to shoulder level, with the palms facing the floor.

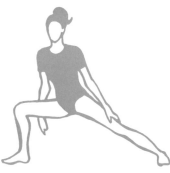
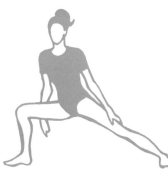

◀ Step 4

Bend your right knee and put it directly above your right heel, the thigh parallel to the floor (aim for a 90° angle at the knee). Extend your body to the right and rest your right forearm on top of your right thigh, body and facing forward.

▶ Step 5

Breathe in; raise your left arm up to the vertical. Reach for the ceiling and take your arm towards your left ear. Feel the stretch along your left side, and feel your right side come closer to your right thigh.

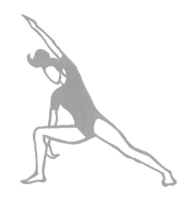

▼ Step 6

Breathe out; place the palm of your right hand on the floor outside your right foot, fingers pointing in the same direction as your right toes. Bring the right side of your body forward, roll the left side back and up towards the ceiling. Feel the diagonal stretch along your left side from outer ankle to fingertips. Hold the posture and breathe normally.

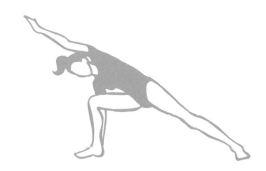

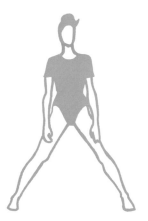

◀ Step 7

Breathe in; straighten your right leg and raise your body up to the vertical. Extend your arms out by your sides at shoulder level. Breathe out; relax your arms down by your sides and turn the toes to point forward.

Step 8

Repeat to the other side from Step 2.

Trikonasana *Triangle*

One of yoga's most recognizable poses, its purpose is to open your chest. Don't be tempted to get down to the floor with the lowered hand or lean on your leg. Your upper back should be parallel to the wall behind you. If you go down too far with the hand, you may drag the upper shoulder forward.

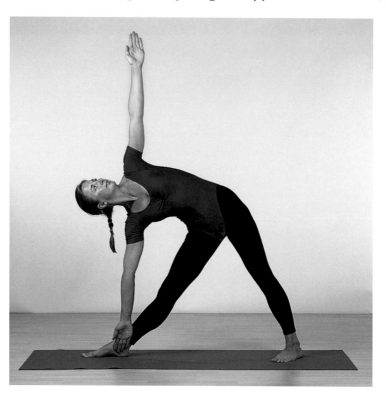

BENEFITS

- Tones the leg and buttock muscles.
- Encourages flexibility in the hips.
- Helps with digestive problems and disorders.
- Opens out the chest.

WATCH OUT!

- Take care if you have knee problems.
- Approach with caution if you have arthritic hips.

THE ASANAS

56

▶ Step 1

Stand with your feet together, flat on the floor, and your body in a straight line, facing forward. Relax your arms by your sides. (See Tadasana, page 48.)

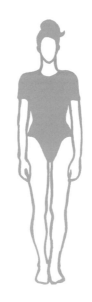

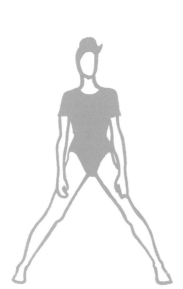

◀ Step 2

Stand with your feet about 1 m (3½ ft) apart.

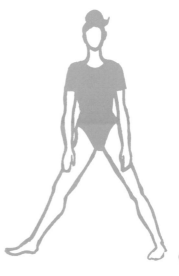

▶ Step 3

Turn your right foot out to a 90° angle and your left foot in to 45° (your right heel is in line with your left instep).

(continued)

▶ Step 4

Breathe in; stretch
your spine up and
raise both your arms
to shoulder level; your
palms face down.

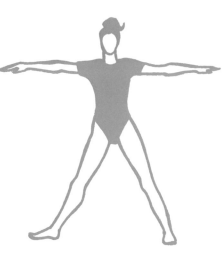

◀ Step 5

Breathe out; extend your right
arm out to the side and bring
your right hand down your right
leg towards the floor, palm
facing forward. Feel the stretch
along the left side of your body.

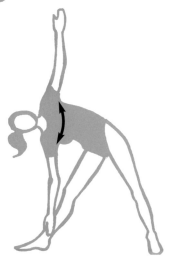

▶ Step 6

Breathe in; raise your left arm
up to the vertical, palm facing
forward. Feel your chest open
and expand.

▶ Step 7

Breathe out; turn your head up towards your left hand. You are aiming to have a straight line from the top hand to the bottom hand.

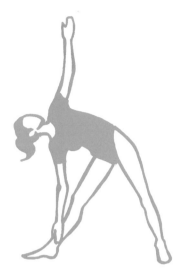

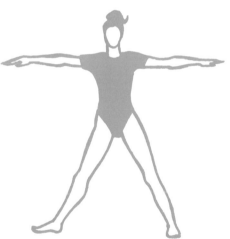

◀ Step 8

Turn your head to look forward and raise your body up to the vertical, arms outstretched at shoulder level.

▶ Step 9

Breathe out; relax your arms down by sides, with your feet now facing forward.

Step 10

Repeat on the other side from Step 3 to the end.

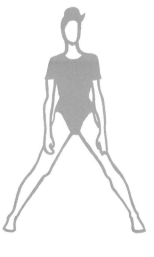

▶ Virabhadrasana I *Warrior 1*

All the standing poses are invigorating, none more so than the Warrior poses. Here, both hips face forward over the front leg – the key to this is ensuring that the back foot is turned in enough to allow the hips to turn fully. Make sure that you lift out of your hips, don't sink into them. If you have blood-pressure problems, do the pose with arms by your sides.

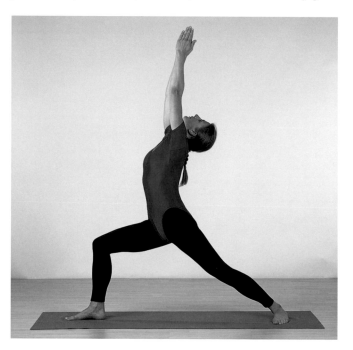

BENEFITS

- Strengthens the ankle and knee joints.
- Helps develop the chest muscles.
- Strengthens the leg muscles.
- Helpful for sciatica sufferers.
- Stimulates and promotes 'inner strength'.

WATCH OUT!

- Take care if you have back, hip or shoulder problems.
- Do not raise arms over head if you have high or low blood pressure.

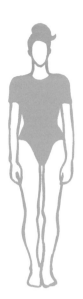

◀ Step 1

Stand with your feet together, flat on the floor, and your body in a straight line, facing forward. Relax your arms by your sides. (See Tadasana, page 48.)

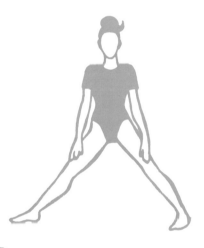

▶ Step 2

Stand with your feet about 1.2 m (4 ft) apart. Turn your right foot out to a 90° angle and your left foot in to 45°; your right heel is in line with your left instep.

◀ Step 3

Breathe out; rotate your hips and turn your body around to the right, so that the front of your body faces in the same direction as your right toes.

(continued)

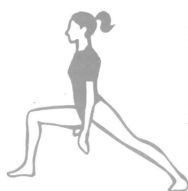

◀ Step 4

Bend your right knee and place it directly over your right heel, right thigh parallel to the floor and right knee pointing directly towards right toes (make a right angle at the right-knee joint). Your left leg is straight. Push the soles of both feet into the floor.

▶ Step 5

Breathe in; raise your arms above your head, keeping them straight and shoulder-width apart with palms facing inwards. Stretch your arms up, fingertips reaching for the ceiling.

▶ Step 6

Breathe out; slowly drop your head back and look up between your palms to the ceiling. Hold the posture and breathe normally. The back of your neck should be soft, not stiff.

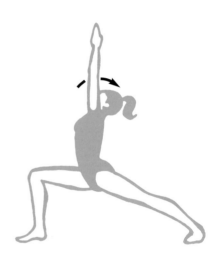

◀ Step 7

Breathe in, raise your head to the vertical; breathe out, straighten your right leg, turn your body to the front, relax your arms by your sides and turn your toes to the front.

Step 8

Keeping your feet wide, repeat to the other side from Step 2.

THE ASANAS

62

Virabhadrasana II
Warrior 2

In this strong standing pose the chest is fully opened to the front. The back foot is turned in about 45°. This means that both hips face forward and they don't turn towards the leading leg. When you turn and look over the outstretched hand, your gaze should be soft and relaxed, not held in a rigid hard stare.

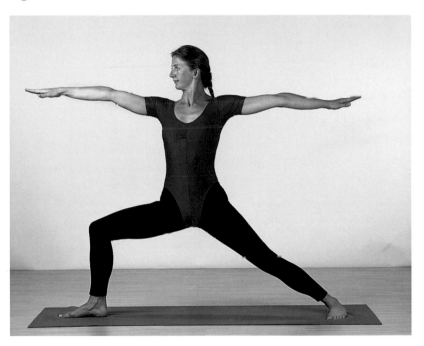

BENEFITS

- Opens and expands the chest.
- Encourages deep breathing.
- Stimulates the abdominal organs.
- Promotes and stimulates 'inner strength'.

WATCH OUT!

- Approach with caution if you have arthritic hips.
- Take care with ankle or knee problems.

▶ Step 1

Stand with your feet
together, flat on the floor,
and your body in a
straight line, facing
forward. Relax your arms
by your sides. (See
Tadasana, page 48.)

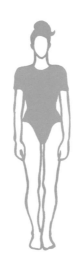

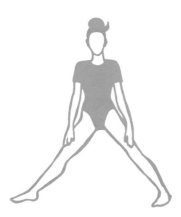

◀ Step 2

Stand with your feet about 1.2 m (4 ft)
apart. Turn your right foot out to a 90°
angle and your left foot in to 45°; your
right heel is in line with your left instep.

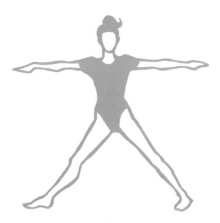

▶ Step 3

Breathe in; extend
your arms out to the
sides at shoulder level,
palms facing the floor
and body facing
forward.

▶ Step 4

Breathe out; bend your right knee and place it directly over your right heel, right thigh parallel to the floor (make a right angle at the right-knee joint). Your left leg is straight. Push the soles of both feet into the floor.

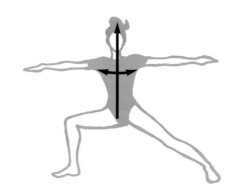

▲ Step 5

Breathe in; extend and stretch your body upwards from the tailbone to the top of the head. Open and expand your body – your front chest and ribcage expand out to the sides. Keep hips and shoulders parallel.

▶ Step 6

Breathe out; turn your head to the right and look to the fingertips of your right hand. Keep your shoulders low and relaxed, body facing forward. Hold the posture and breathe normally.

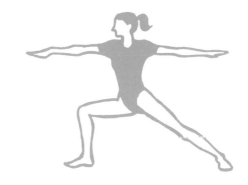

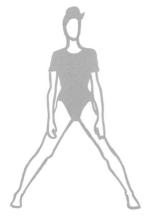

◀ Step 7

Breathe in; straighten your right leg. Breathe out, turn your head and toes to face the front again; relax your arms by your sides.

Step 8

Keeping your feet wide, repeat to the other side from Step 2.

▶ Ardha chandrasana
Half moon

This balance pose strengthens the legs and lower spine. The body weight is taken by the supporting leg and hip, not the hand on the floor. This hand is to help control your balance.

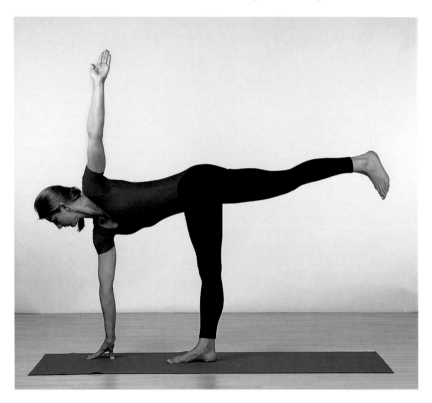

THE ASANAS

66

BENEFITS

- Encourages mobility in the hips.
- Opens and expands the front of the body.
- Increases the circulation to the lower half of the body.

WATCH OUT!

- Avoid if you have arthritic hips.
- If unsteady, practise with your back against a wall.

◄ Step 1

Stand with your feet together, flat on the floor, and your body in a straight line, facing forward. Relax your arms by your sides. (See Tadasana, page 48.)

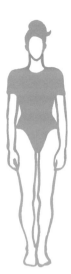

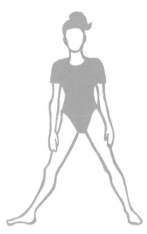

◄ Step 2

Stand with your feet about 1 m (3¼ ft) apart. Turn your right foot out to a 90° angle and your left foot in to 45°; your right heel is in line with your left instep.

Step 3

Breathe in; raise your arms out to shoulder level, palms facing the floor. Bring your right hand down towards your right foot. Relax your left arm and hand along your left side; your body faces forward.

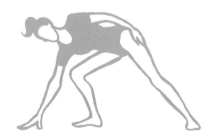

◄ Step 4

Bend your right knee and place your right fingertips on the floor, 30 cm (1 ft) in front of your right foot. Your body faces forward, and your face is looking straight ahead. (continued)

▶ Step 5

Breathe in; raise your left leg straight up to the horizontal in line with your left hip; your toes and knee face forward. Push your left heel away from your body and stretch your left leg. At the same time, straighten your right leg.

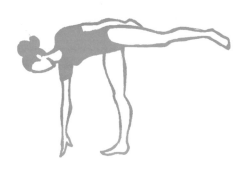

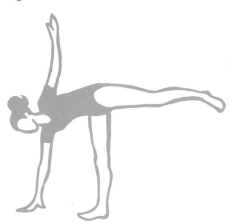

◀ Step 6

Breathe out; straighten your right arm. Your right hand does not bear any weight – it is simply for balance. Raise your left arm up to the vertical, pushing your fingertips up to the ceiling with your palm facing forward (your left arm is in line with your right arm). Bring the right side of your body forward, rolling the left side back and up to the ceiling. Feel the front of your body open and expand. Hold the posture and breathe normally.

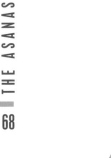

◀ Step 7

Bend your right knee and stretch your left leg back to put the sole of your left foot on the floor. Straighten both legs. Breathe in; raise your body to the vertical, arms outstretched at shoulder level. Breathe out; relax your arms down by your sides, feet facing forward.

Step 8

Repeat the pose to the other side from Step 2.

Uttanasana
Standing forward bend

When attempting this pose at first, you may find that your
palms do not touch the floor. If this is the case you can place
them around your ankles or on the backs of your legs,
whichever is more comfortable.

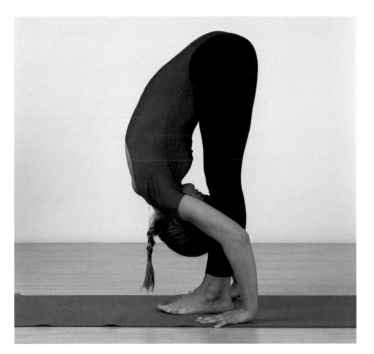

BENEFITS

- Improves upper-body circulation.
- Calms yet energizes the body.
- Stimulates and tones the abdominal
organs.
- Tones the leg muscles.

WATCH OUT!

- Avoid if you have eye
problems.
- Avoid if you have
blood-pressure
problems.
- Take care if you
have lower-back pain.

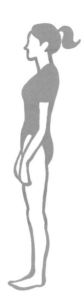

◄ Step 1

Stand with your feet together, flat on the floor, and your body in a straight line, facing forward. Relax your arms by your sides. (See Tadasana, page 48.)

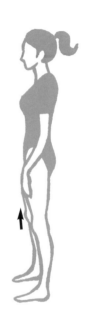

► Step 2

Take feet hip-width apart, feet parallel, toes pointing forward. Pull your kneecaps up (feel legs strengthen and stretch).

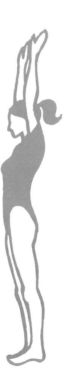

◄ Step 3

Breathe in; stretch your spine upwards from your tailbone to the top of your head and raise your arms straight above your head, shoulder-width apart, the palms facing forward.

▶ Step 4

Breathe out; extend your body and arms forward, hingeing from the hips. Lead with your chest (to flatten the back) and bring your chest and abdomen down onto the front of your thighs; place your forehead on your shins.

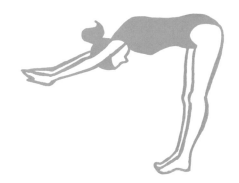

▼ Step 5

Place the palms of your hands down onto the floor beside your feet, fingers pointing forward. Gently push the palms into the floor and bring the front of your body close in to the front of the legs, with the top of your head facing the floor.

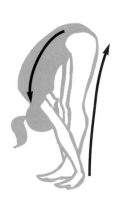

◀ Step 6

Hold the posture and breathe normally. Feel the stretch up your legs, from your heels to your buttock bones, and feel your spine extending downwards from your tailbone to the top of your head.

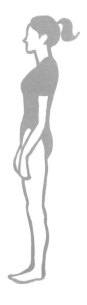

▶ Step 7

To come out: bend your knees, breathe in and raise your body and arms to the vertical. Breathe out, lower your arms down by your sides and straighten your legs.

▶ Parsvottanasana
Sideways forward bend

This is a good posture for keeping hips loose and flexible as well as for toning the abdominal organs that get a good squeeze when you take your head towards your knees. Don't let your shoulders fall forwards. Keep shoulder blades pulled back to encourage deep breathing.

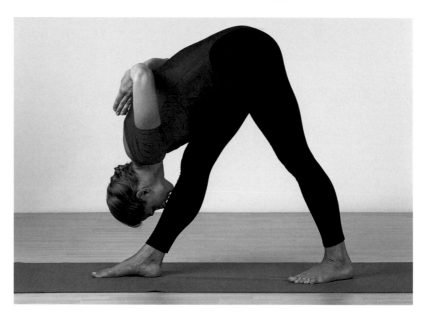

BENEFITS

- Brings about flexibility in the wrists, shoulders and hips.
- Relieves leg stiffness.
- Stimulates and tones the abdominal organs.
- Helps correct rounded shoulders.

WATCH OUT!

- Avoid if you have eye problems.
- Avoid if you have blood-pressure problems.
- Take care if you have arthritic hips, shoulders or wrists.

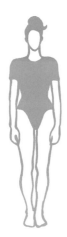

◀ Step 1

Stand with your feet together, flat on the floor, and your body in a straight line, facing forward. Relax your arms by your sides. (See Tadasana, page 48.)

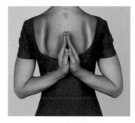

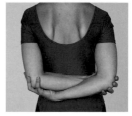

▶ Step 2

Bring the palms of your hands together into a prayer position (Namaste) behind your back, the hands in line with the shoulder blades. The outside edges of your little fingers should be in contact with your spine and your fingers pointed to the ceiling (right, top).
If this is too difficult, bend your arms at the elbows behind your back and take hold of your right elbow with your left hand, and your left elbow with your right (right, bottom).

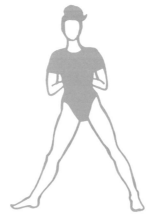

▶ Step 3

Stand with your feet 1 m (about 3 - 3½ ft) apart. Turn your right foot out to a 90° angle and your left foot in to 45°; your right heel should be in line with your left instep.

(continued)

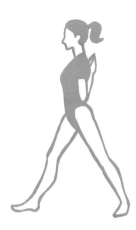

◀ Step 4

Rotate your body from the hips to turn round to the right, so that the front of your body faces forward in the same direction as your right toes.

Step 5

Breathe in; stretch your spine up from your tailbone to the top of your head. Open and expand the body.

▶ Step 6

Breathe out; extend your body forward from the hips, leading with chin (to flatten the back), and stretch the body down along the right leg. Aim to place your abdomen and chest on your right thigh, and your forehead on your right shin. Lengthen spine your and the back of your neck down towards the floor, with the top of your head facing the floor; tuck your chin in. Stretch your elbows up to the ceiling, keeping your hands in Namaste. Hold the posture, breathing normally. On each out-breath, stretch and extend your body further down into the posture. Push your tailbone up towards the ceiling, and widen the buttocks.

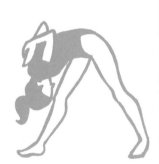

▶ Step 7

Breathe in; raise your head and body to the vertical; breathe out, turn your body to the front, release the hands and relax your arms down by your sides, turning your toes to point forward.

Step 8

Repeat the pose to the other side from Step 2.

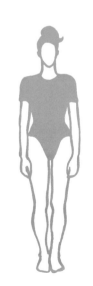

Prasarita padottanasana
Wide-leg forward bend

Some people are very good at bending forward from the hip joints, others find it hard work. Don't compare, just keep working in the pose. With your head down towards the floor, blood flows into your upper body and brain, refreshing all the organs and glands. This is one of the easier ways of doing an upside down pose.

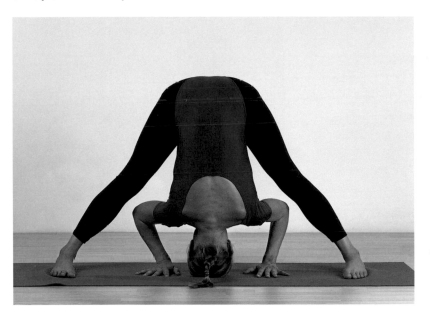

BENEFITS

- Opens and expands the chest and hips.
- Increases circulation in the upper body.
- Stretches the leg and thigh muscles.
- Aids digestion.

WATCH OUT!

- Avoid forward bends if you have eye problems.
- Do not attempt if you have high or low blood pressure.
- Go slowly, especially if you have a slipped disc or other back problems.
- Take care if you have head, ear or neck problems.

▶ Step 1

Stand with your feet together, flat on the floor, and your body in a straight line, facing forward. Relax your arms by your sides. (See Tadasana, page 48.)

▼ Step 2

Take your feet 1.4 m (4½ ft) apart, keeping them parallel, with your toes pointing forward. Pull your kneecaps up and lift your insteps (feel your legs strengthen).

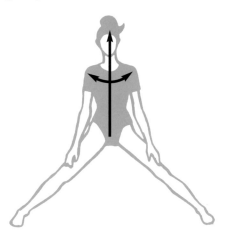

◀ Step 3

Breathe in; extend your spine upwards from your tailbone to the top of your head. Lift and open the front of your body. Tuck your tailbone under and forwards.

▶ Step 4

Breathe out; extend your body forward, hingeing at the hips. Lead with your chest to flatten your back, and bring your body to the horizontal, parallel with the floor. Place your palms on the floor directly below your shoulders with your arms straight and fingers pointing forward.

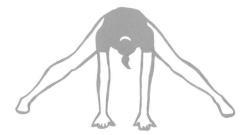

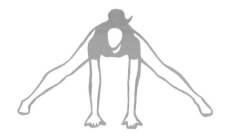

Breathe in; raise your head and look forward. Take your hands back in line with your feet, your palms on floor, shoulder-width apart and your fingers point forward.

▶ Step 6

Breathe out; bend your elbows back below your body (making right angles with your arms). Extend your body and spine downwards and bring the top of your head down onto the floor, below your body. Push your palms into the floor, keeping your elbows bent, then lift your shoulders and push your tailbone up to the ceiling (feel your back extending). Breathe normally. On each out-breath stretch and extend your body further down into the posture.

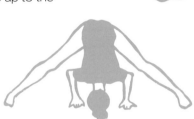

▶ Step 7

Breathe in, raise your head and body to the horizontal with your arms straight and palms on the floor below your shoulders. Breathe out, move your feet closer by pointing in your toes then heels until your feet are together. Breathe in, raise your body and head to the vertical; breathe out, move your toes and heels to bring your feet together, and relax your arms down by your sides.

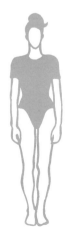

STANDING POSTURES

77

Dandasana *Rod or Staff*

To make sure you are seated on your sitting bones, use your hands to separate each buttock. (To find your sitting bones, slide the flats of your hands, palms down, beneath your buttocks – you should feel the bony bits sticking into the backs of your hands.) Whereas in Tadasana (mountain pose) the weight of the body is spread across the soles of the feet, in Dandasana it is spread across the sitting bones.

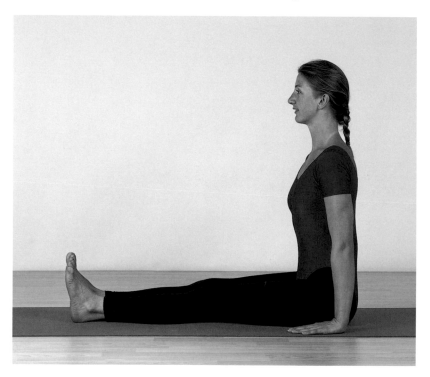

BENEFITS

- Strengthens leg muscles.
- Opens the front of the chest.
- Improves whole-body posture.
- Brings about body awareness.

▶ Step 1

Sit tall on your buttock bones, your legs outstretched in front of you, relaxing your arms by your sides.

Step 2

Bring your legs together so the inner-ankle bones and inner-knee joints are touching. (If you find this difficult, leave your legs slightly apart.)

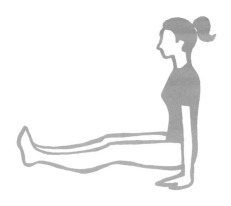

◀ Step 3

Push your heels away from your body, your toes pointing upward. Breathe in; straighten and stretch up through your spine, from your tailbone to the top of your head. Breathe out; relax your shoulders down, and open and expand the front of your body, keeping your spine straight.

▶ Step 4

Relax your arms by your sides with your palms resting on the floor beside your hips, and fingers pointing forward.

Step 5

Lengthen the back of your neck by lowering your chin slightly; balance your head evenly over your spine, face looking forward. Maintain a straight upright posture, hold and breathe normally.

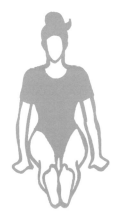

▶ Virasana *Hero*

When you first practise this pose, you may find you are not flexible enough to rest your buttocks on the floor between your feet. Place a folded blanket or two beneath you, and rest the buttocks on the blankets.

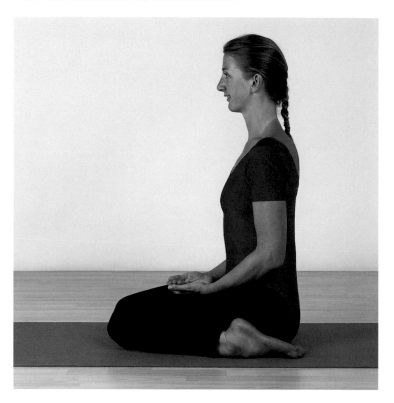

BENEFITS

- Opens the chest and encourages deep breathing.
- Helpful for respiratory problems.
- Stimulates the leg muscles.
- Beneficial for flat feet.
- Calms the whole body.

WATCH OUT!

- Do not practise if you have knee or hip problems.
- Do not practise if you have varicose veins.

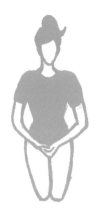

◀ Step 1

Kneel, with your spine straight and body facing forward. Bring your thighs together so that the inner knee joints and ankle bones are touching. The tops of your feet are on floor, toes pointing back.

Step 2

Put your buttocks onto your heels. Put your palms onto the floor beside your hips. Relax your shoulders and arms.

▶ Step 3

Keeping your knees together, take your feet apart and with your hands, roll both calf muscles out to sides and down to floor. Put your feet at the outside of your buttocks; your toes point back and the soles of your feet face the ceiling. Sit between your feet.

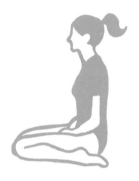

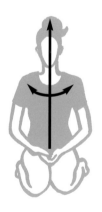

◀ Step 4

Breathe in; stretch your spine up, from your tailbone to the top of your head. Open and expand the front of your body, face looking straight ahead. Rest your hands on the front of your thighs. Relax your arms and shoulders.

Step 5

Breathe out; keeping your thighs together, roll the front thigh muscles out to the sides. The front of your thighs face the ceiling, and your shins rest on the floor.

Step 6

Hold the posture and breathe normally. Stretch your body up, keeping your buttocks firmly on the floor.

Baddha konasana
Cobbler

This pose is very good for the organs in the pelvic area, keeping healthy the kidneys and bladder, and the prostate in men. It is especially good for women, regulating menstrual cycles and keeping the ovaries functioning properly.

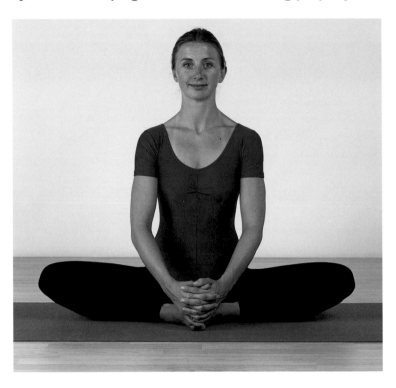

BENEFITS

- Stimulates the abdominal organs.
- Relieves lower-back pain.
- Helps urinary-related and menstrual problems.
- Strengthens the leg muscles.

WATCH OUT!

- Avoid if you suffer severe knee problems.
- Never push the knees down with the hands.

◀ Step 1

Sit on both buttock bones, your spine straight, body facing forward and shoulders parallel. Bring your legs together, outstretched in front of your body. Relax your arms down by your sides. (See Dandasana, page 78.)

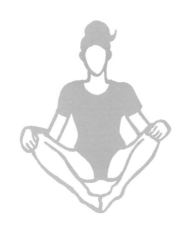

▶ Step 2

Bend your knees out to the sides and bring the soles of your feet together in front of your body.

◀ Step 3

Clasp your hands, interlinking your fingers around the toes of both feet, and draw your heels in towards your crotch. The outside edges of both your feet and your little toes remain on the floor.

▲ Step 4

Breathe in; stretch your spine upwards from your tailbone to the top of your head. Open and stretch up the front of your body, keeping your shoulders relaxed and parallel.

(continued)

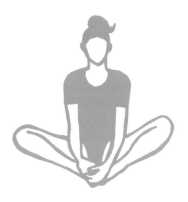

◀ Step 5

Breathe out; push your knees out to each side, rolling your inner-calf and thigh muscles up towards the ceiling. Feel your thighs easing out from your hip joints.

▶ Step 6

Hold the posture, keeping your spine straight and stretching your body upwards. On every out-breath, extend your knees further out to each side; aim to bring the outsides of your legs and knees down onto the floor.

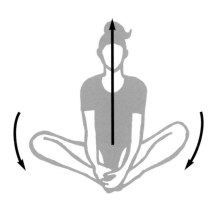

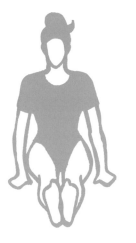

◀ Step 7

Take your hands to the outsides of your knees, and keep your legs bent and bring them together, in towards body. Breathe out; stretch your legs in front and relax your arms by your sides.

THE ASANAS

84

Sukhasana *Easy pose*

The easiest of all cross-legged positions, Sukhasana allows the spine to be straight, making it suitable for short meditation periods (with hands resting on knees). If your knees are high, you will find it uncomfortable to sit in this position for long periods. The lower the knees, the more comfortable it is.

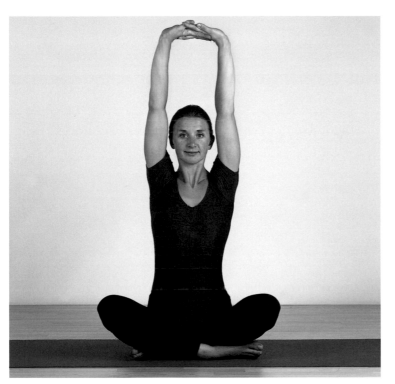

BENEFITS

- Strengthens the spine.
- Encourages deep breathing.
- Tones the nervous system.
- Induces calmness in the body.

WATCH OUT!

- Take care if you have a weak back.
- Never push the knees down with the hands.

▶ Step 1

Sit on both buttock bones, your spine straight, body facing forward and shoulders parallel. Bring your legs together, outstretched in front of your body. Relax your arms down by your sides. (See Dandasana, page 78.)

Step 2

Bend your knees out to the sides.

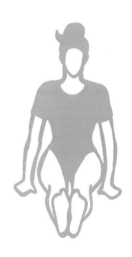

▶ Step 3

Place the top of your right foot onto the floor in front of your left shin; the sole of your right foot rolls up towards the ceiling. Place the top of your left foot on the floor at the inside of your right thigh; the sole of your left foot rolls up towards the ceiling.

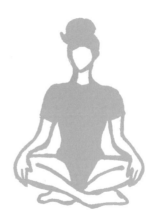

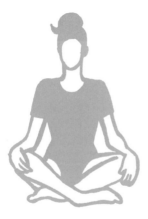

◀ Step 4

Bring your knees in closer together, legs crossed in front of your body (the tops of your feet and your buttocks stay on the floor). Relax your legs down to floor. Place your palms on your knees with the fingers gently curved; relax your arms and shoulders.

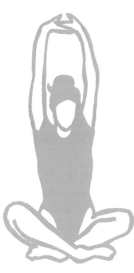

◄ Step 5

Breathe in; interlock your fingers. Turn your palms outwards as you raise your arms above your head.

Step 6

Hold the posture and breathe normally. Extend your body upwards on each in-breath.

► Step 7

Uncross your legs and stretch them out in front; unclasp your hands and relax your arms by your sides.

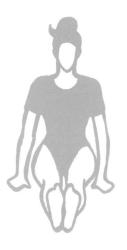

Step 8

Repeat the posture to the other side, placing your left foot in front of your right shin.

Upavista konasana
Seated wide-leg forward bend

As with all forward bends, the bending should come from the hips, not the upper back. You should sit on your sitting bones, pressing your heels away from you and the backs of your knees to the floor. Tight hips and tight hamstrings might make this more difficult. The muscles on the insides of the thighs get a good stretch.

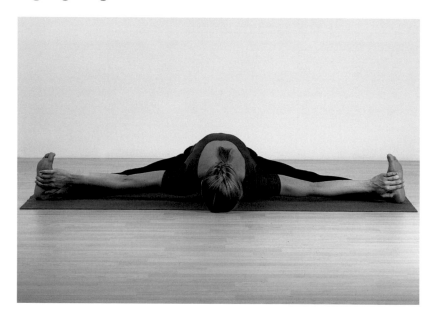

BENEFITS

- Improves pelvic circulation.
- Stretches the hamstrings.
- Helps gynaecological and menstrual problems.
- Loosens the hip joints.
- Can relieve or release sciatic pain.
- Helpful for hernia problems.

WATCH OUT!

- Take care if you have back problems.
- Do not bounce into or in the posture.
- Take care if you have tight hamstring muscles.

▶ Step 1

Sit on both buttock bones, your spine straight, body facing forward and shoulders parallel. Bring your legs together, outstretched in front of your body. Relax your arms down by your sides. (See Dandasana, page 78.)

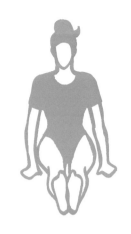

▼ Step 2

Spread your legs wide apart, about 1.25 m (4 ft); each of your legs should be the same distance apart from your body. Push your heels away from your body; your toes point up to the ceiling.

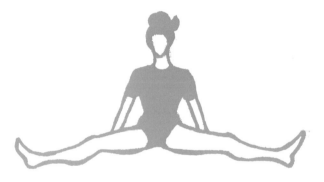

▼ Step 3

Keeping your buttocks on the floor, hinge your body forward from the hips and stretch your arms down the insides of your legs. Place your palms around your feet, or at any point that is comfortable on inside of your legs.

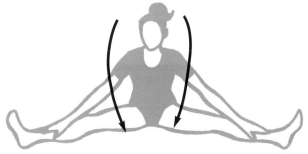

(continued)

▶ Step 4

Breathe in; lift and open the front of the body,
pulling abdomen muscles in and up. Stretch
and lengthen spine from tailbone to top of
head; pull in and concave the lower back.

▼ Step 5

Breathe out; extend and stretch your body forward from
the hips, leading with the chest to flatten the back. Keep
both buttocks on the floor, aiming to bring your abdomen,
chest and chin down onto the floor between your legs.

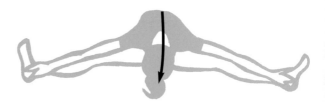

Step 6

Breathe normally; on each out-breath extend
and stretch your body further forward into the
posture. Lengthen out your spine and the back
of the neck. Relax head; push the top of your
head away from your body.

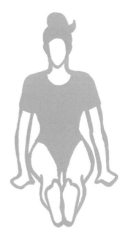

▶ Step 7

To come out: breathe in, raise your body to the
vertical; breathe out, relax your arms by your
sides and bring your legs together outstretched
in front of your body.

THE ASANAS

Paschimottanasana
Seated forward bend

Forward bends are calming and quietening poses. In the full
pose the head lies lower than the spine (you should be
practically folded in two) and both heart and abdominal
organs get a good massage. Some people find it very
difficult to bend forward from the hips, but go as far as you
can. Do not be tempted to try to get your head down
towards the legs by bending the upper spine.

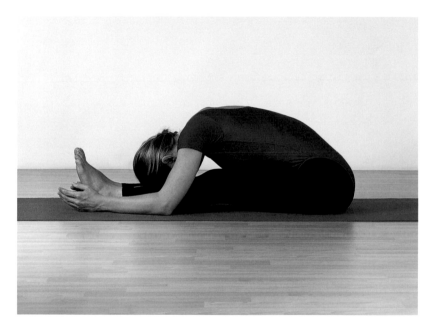

BENEFITS

- An excellent stretch for the whole of the
back of the body.
- Tones the kidneys and abdominal organs.
- Improves digestion and circulation.
- Induces calmness in the body.

WATCH OUT!

- Take care if you
have back problems
or sciatica.
- Do not bounce in
the posture.

▶ Step 1

Sit on both buttock bones, your spine straight, body facing forward and shoulders parallel. Bring your legs together, outstretched in front of your body. Relax your arms down by your sides. (See Dandasana, page 78.)

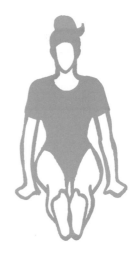

▼ Step 2

Extend your body forward, hingeing at the hips; keep your head up to flatten your back, and bring your hands down to your feet. Place your palms around outside of your feet, or in any position that is comfortable on outside of your legs. Relax your arms.

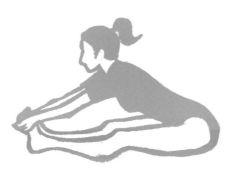

Step 3

Push heels away from body, letting toes point to the ceiling.

Step 4

Breathe in; stretch and lengthen your spine from your tailbone to the top of your head. Pull your abdomen muscles in and up; open and extend your body.

▼ Step 5

Breathe out; extend your body forward, leading with your chin. Aim to bring your hips, abdomen and chest down onto the front of your thighs and to put your forehead on your shins. Push the top of your head away from your body, lengthening your spine and the back of your neck. Relax your head and shoulders. Relax your arms on the floor by your sides.

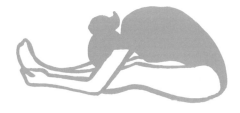

Step 6

Hold the posture and breathe normally. On each out-breath stretch and extend your body further forward, aiming to rest the whole of the front of the body down onto the legs. Keep your back flat.

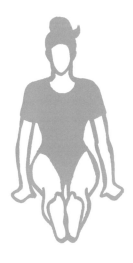

◄ Step 7

Breathe in, raise your body and head to the vertical; breathe out, relax your arms by your sides; relax your legs.

▶ Hamsasana *Swan*

In this pose, the head rests lightly on the floor and the heart is higher than the head. This allows fresh blood to flow into the upper chest and brain. Hamasana also gives the spine a good stretch.

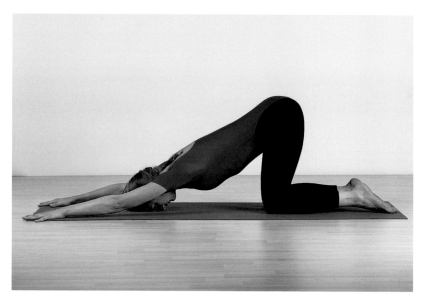

BENEFITS

- Strengthens the back and arm muscles.
- Stretches the spine.
- Tones the buttock muscles.
- Helps lower-back pain.

WATCH OUT!

- Be careful if you have knee problems.
- Take care if you have back problems.

THE ASANAS

94

◄ Step 1

From a kneeling position, come up onto your hands and knees.

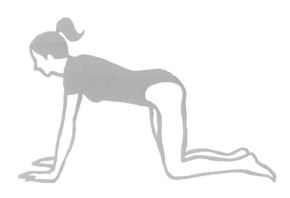

► Step 2

Put your hands, palms-down, directly below your shoulders; your arms are straight, your fingers point forward. Place your knees directly below your hips; your shins and the tops of your feet rest on the floor, toes pointing back. Your trunk is parallel to the floor.

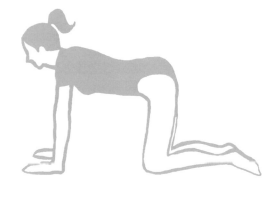

◄ Step 3

Breathe in; raise your head and look forward, open and expand the front of your chest; pull in and make your lower back concave.

(continued)

▼ Step 4

Breathe out; pulling in your lower back, push
your tailbone back and up towards ceiling;
simultaneously walk your palms forward in front
of your body, shoulder-width apart. Straightening
your arms, extend and lower your body down
towards the floor; put your head on the floor
between your arms (feel your spine lengthen).
Relax your neck and head.

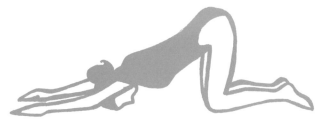

Step 5

Hold the posture and breathe normally.

▶ Step 6

Push your buttocks back onto your heels, and
allow your arms and hands to slide back to your
sides. Breathe in; raise your body and head to
the vertical. Breathe out.

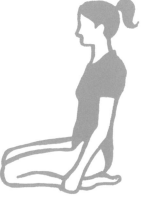

Gomukhasana *Cow face*

Beginners may find this seated pose demanding. If you can't manage to clasp your hands behind your back, hold a belt or sock in the top hand and grasp it with the lower hand instead. If kneeling is too difficult, rest your buttocks on your heels, with the tops of your feet on the floor and toes pointing back, to complete the pose.

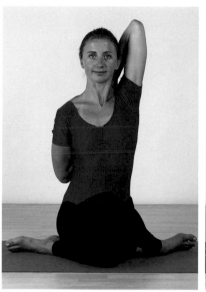 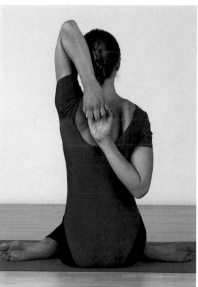

BENEFITS

- Opens and expands the front of the body.
- Helpful for respiratory problems.
- Encourages deep breathing.
- Strengthens arm and back muscles.
- Helps rounded shoulders and improves posture.
- Eases bursitis.

WATCH OUT!

- Take care if you have an abdominal complaint.
- Approach this posture with care if you suffer from back or knee problems.

▶ Step 1

Sit tall on both buttock bones, your spine straight, body facing forward and legs out-stretched in front of your body, as in Dandasana (see page 78).

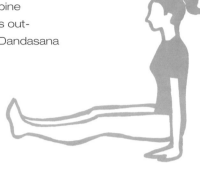

◀ Step 2

Bend your left leg at the knee and place the top of your left foot below your right buttock. Bend your right leg at the knee, and place the bottom of your right thigh onto the top of your left thigh, placing your right knee directly above your left knee. Rest the tops of both feet on the floor, toes pointing backwards; bring your feet close in to your buttocks.

Step 3

Sit your buttocks onto your heels, your body straight and extending upwards, facing forward. Relax your arms by your sides.

Step 4

Breathe in; raise your left arm out in front of your body at shoulder level, arm straight and palm facing upwards. Raise the arm vertically.

▶ Step 5

Bend your left arm at the elbow and drop your left hand and arm down your back; you are aiming to clasp your hands together at the shoulder blades.

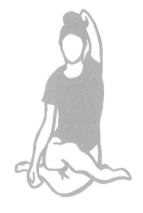

▼ Step 6

Breathe out; bend your right arm at the elbow
and place it up behind your body, bringing the
back of your hand up between your shoulder
blades; bring your right elbow close in towards
your body. (Your left arm, behind your head,
points up to the ceiling; your right elbow, behind
your body, points down to the floor. See the
back, side and front views of the posture.)

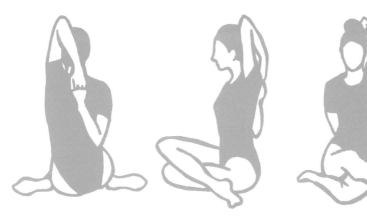

Step 7

Extend and open out the front of your body,
keeping your head, shoulders and face relaxed.
Hold the pose and breathe normally.

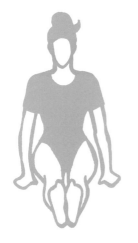

◀ Step 8

To come out of the posture: release your hands
and bring your arms down by your sides.
Release your legs by pushing your palms down
into the floor at the sides of your body. Lift your
buttocks off the floor, release your right leg and
straighten it out in front of your body. Release
your left leg and straighten it out in front of your
body. Relax your arms by your sides.

Step 9

Repeat the pose to the other side, using the
opposite limbs throughout.

▶ Balasana *Pose of a child*

In this posture, it is important that the back of the body, the spine, the neck and the head are all relaxed. There should be no strain. If your forehead doesn't extend to the floor, put a folded blanket in front of your knees to rest your forehead on. Likewise, place a blanket on your heels if your buttocks cannot come down to rest between the heels.

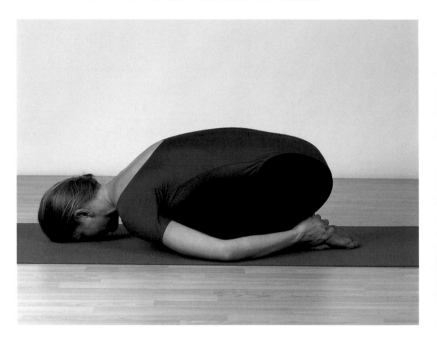

BENEFITS

- Improves circulation to the head and face.
- Eases tension in the back and legs.
- Stretches the spine.
- Encourages the whole body to relax.

WATCH OUT!

- Take care if you have knee problems.

▶ Step 1

Come into a kneeling
position on the floor.
Place your buttocks
on your heels, the
spine straight, body
facing forward and
your arms relaxed by
your sides.

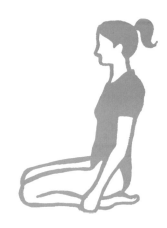

Step 2

Bring your legs together, the inner-ankle bones
and the inner-knee joints touching. The tops of
your feet rest on the floor, toes pointing forward
and the front of your thighs facing the ceiling.

Step 3

Breathe in; stretch your spine upwards from
your tailbone to the top of your head. Open and
expand the front of your body.

▶ Step 4

Breathe out; extend
your body forward,
hinging at the hips;
lead with your chin to
flatten your back.
Keep both buttocks
on your heels and
place your forehead
on the floor in front of
your knees (let front of
your body rest on top
of your thighs).

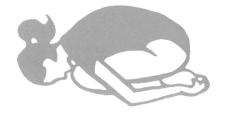

▲ Step 5

Place palms of your hands on the soles of your
feet. Relax your back, neck and head. Hold the
posture and breathe normally.

Savasana *Corpse*

Savasana is the classic lying-down posture. If your body is too uncomfortable lying with the legs outstretched, or you have backache or back problems, bend your knees up and place the soles of your feet on the ground – not too close or too far from the buttocks – so that the whole of your spine is relaxed on the floor. Your feet should be hip-width apart and your toes pointing forward. Relax your lower back down onto the floor.

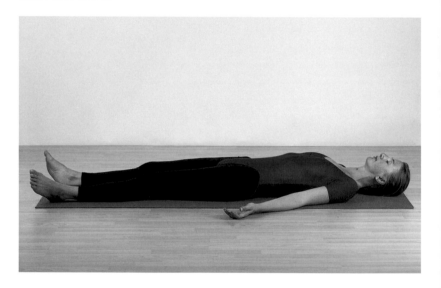

BENEFITS

- Eases tension in the muscles.
- Calms the nervous system.
- Can benefit heart problems.

WATCH OUT!

- Approach with caution if you have back problems.

THE ASANAS

▼ Step 1

Lie with your back flat on floor and your body in
a straight line, facing the ceiling. Relax your arms
by your sides, palms up. Close your eyes.

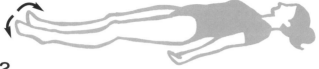

▲ Step 2

Take your feet hip-width apart; your feet fall out
to the sides. Relax your lower back. Push your
shoulders down away from your ears, and
stretch out the back of your neck.

Step 3

Soften and relax your facial muscles. Relax your
throat and the front of your neck. Swallow a few
times; rest your tongue loosely behind your
upper teeth; your chin is pointing to your feet.

▶ Step 4

Relax your pelvis,
abdomen and
diaphragm. Open and
expand your ribs and the
front of your chest.
Spread your collarbones
out to the sides (feel the
front of your body open).
Relax the entire back of
your body down into the floor, letting its
weight be supported by the floor. Your body
is still and motionless.

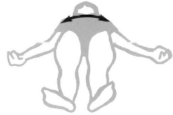

Step 5

Focus your attention on your breath: breathe through both nostrils and let
your breathing slow down and become quiet. On each out-breath let the
back of your body relax deeper into the floor; release and let go of any
physical, mental and emotional tension.

▶ Anantasana
Sideways hand–big toe

This pose tones the pelvic area and relaxes the hamstrings and inner-thigh muscles. Make sure your hips are in line, one directly above the other; otherwise you lose the stretch. If you find it hard to balance, bend the lower leg slightly.

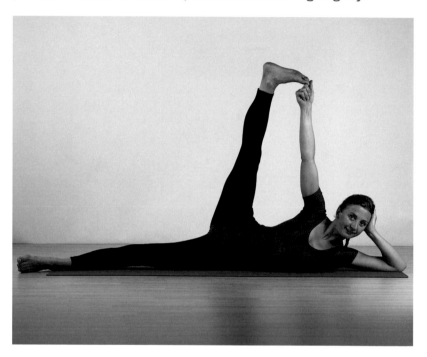

BENEFITS

- Stimulates the leg muscles.
- Stretches the hamstrings.
- Increases mobility in the hips.
- Helpful for back pain.
- Tones the pelvic area.
- Helps prevent hernia problems.

WATCH OUT!

- Avoid if you have arthritis in your hips.
- Take care if you have problems or arthritis in wrists or shoulders.

▼ Step 1

Lie with your back flat on floor and your body in
a straight line. Relax your arms by your sides;
your palms face the ceiling.

▼ Step 2

Turn and rest your left side on the floor. Bring
your feet and legs together, with legs straight.
Bend your left arm at the elbow so that your
upper arm is on the floor behind and beyond
your head, in line with your body, and your elbow
points away from your body. Support your head
above your ear with the palm of your left hand.

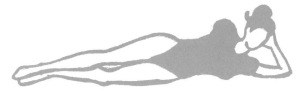

Step 3

Bring the left side of your body into a straight line
from elbow to heel. Push your left armpit down
into the floor; your body weight is resting on your
left side.

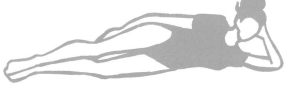

▲ Step 4

Put your right arm and hand along the right side
of your body.

(continued)

▶ Step 5

Breathe in; bend your right knee up towards your face. Bring your right arm and hand to the inside of your right leg, and hook the index finger and thumb of your right hand around your right big toe.

▶ Step 6

Breathe out; rotate your right hip and leg up towards the ceiling and, holding your right big toe with your index finger and thumb, stretch your right leg and arm up to the vertical. Straighten your right leg and push your heel away from your body. Straighten your right arm. Hold the posture and breathe normally.

▼ Step 7

Release your right big toe, bend your right knee down towards your face. Stretch your right leg out and put it on top of your left. Release your left arm from below your body. Turn and rest the back of your body on the floor. Relax your arms by the sides, palms facing the ceiling.

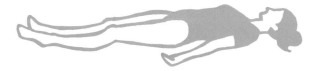

Step 8

Repeat on the right side from Step 1.

Chaturanga dandasana
Plank

This pose requires upper-body strength but is a very good weight-bearing exercise. Your body should be held in a straight line. Don't stick your bottom in the air or drop your head out of alignment. It forms part of the sixth of the twelve poses of Surya Namaskar (the Salutation to the Sun) and one that is frequently omitted by lowering straight to the floor, without lowering into Chaturanga dandasana (the Plank pose) beforehand.

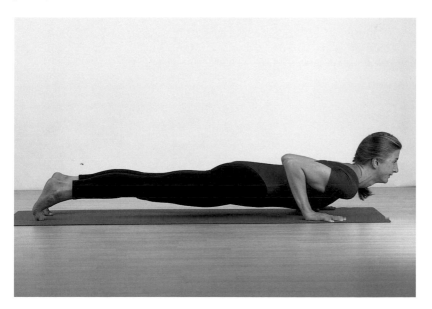

BENEFITS

- Strengthens the shoulders, arms and wrists.
- Tones the abdomen.
- Strengthens the leg muscles.
- Helpful for back pain.

WATCH OUT!

- Avoid if you have back problems.
- Avoid if you have arthritic hips, wrists or shoulders.

▼ Step 1

Lie with your front flat on the floor, your body in a
straight line and legs together. Rest your chin on
the floor; your face looks straight ahead. Relax
your arms by sides, palms facing the ceiling.

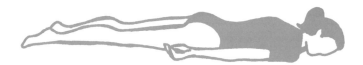

▼ Step 2

Take legs 30 cm (1 ft) apart. Tuck toes under
and push heels away from body. Pull kneecaps
up and stretch out backs of legs.

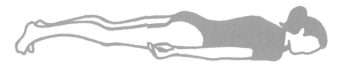

▼ Step 3

Bend your elbows and place your palms on the
floor at either side of your chest, your fingers
spread wide and point forward. Bring your
elbows close in, in line with your shoulders.

▼ Step 4

Breathe in; raise your chin and head, and look straight ahead.

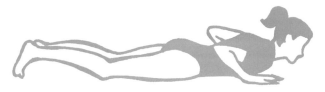

▼ Step 5

Breathe out; push your body weight onto your palms and toes and raise a few inches off the floor, keeping your body parallel with the floor and face forward. Push your shoulders up and back towards your waist. Keeping your toes on the floor, push the backs of your legs up towards the ceiling. Feel your whole body strong, balancing its weight on palms and toes. Hold the posture and breathe normally.

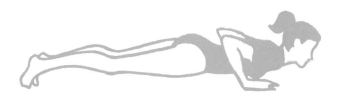

▼ Step 6

Breathe out; lower your front onto the floor. Relax your arms by your sides, palms face up. Rest one side of your head on the floor; relax the front of your body into the floor.

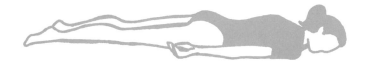

Matsyasana *Fish*

Matsyasana is a backbend. Take care not to put too much pressure on the crown of the head: most of the weight is taken by the elbows and the buttocks. The stretch over the front of the stomach tones the abdominal organs and can help relieve constipation. The stretch over the front of the neck and that regulates the functioning of the thyroid gland, and the open chest encourages deep breathing.

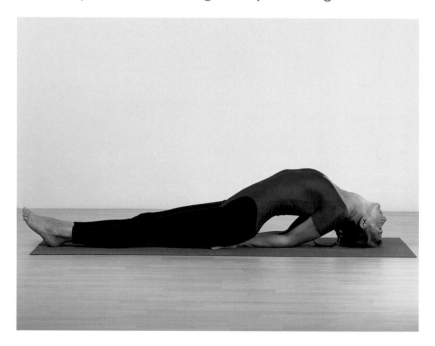

BENEFITS

- Helps respiratory problems.
- Eases tension in the neck area.
- Opens the chest.
- Tones the heart.
- Eases upper-body congestion.
- Stimulates the thyroid and para-thyroid glands.

WATCH OUT!

- Approach with caution if you have back problems.
- Take care if you have neck or shoulder problems.

THE ASANAS

110

▼ Step 1

Lie with your back flat on the floor, your body in
a straight line, and your legs together. Relax your
arms by your sides with palms facing the floor.

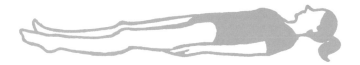

▼ Step 2

Slide your right arm and hand under the right
side of your body, and your left arm and hand
under the left side. Palms rest on the floor below
your buttocks, fingers point towards your feet.

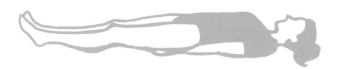

▼ Step 3

Breathe in; raise your head, shoulders, upper
arms and body up off the floor (coming up to
rest on your forearms and palms). Keep your
buttocks and legs on the floor. Push the front of
your body forward and up towards the ceiling;
open and expand the front of the chest.

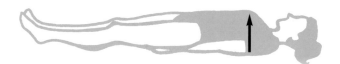

(continued)

▼ Step 4

Breathe out; push your elbows down into the floor, curve your body back and the lower top of your head onto the floor. Arch your back and raise the front chest further up. Push your heels away from the body, stretching.

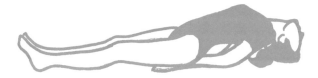

▼ Step 5

If you are more advanced, you can release your arms and hands from below your body and bring hands into Namaste (prayer position) at front of your chest: place the heels of your hands at the middle of your chest, fingers pointing up to the ceiling. Hold the posture, arching the back and breathing normally.

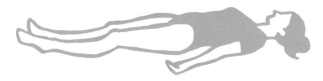

▼ Step 6

Bring your arms down by your sides. Breathe out; push your palms down into the floor and slide the back of your head onto the floor, taking care not to strain your neck. Relax your back down onto the floor (lowering from top to bottom of the spine). Relax your arms by your sides, palms facing the ceiling. Relax the whole of the back of the body down onto the floor.

THE ASANAS

Supta padangusthasana
Lying down hand–big toe

This is a great pose for the legs and hips. The legs benefit from the increased circulation of the blood and the hips become more flexible. It also relieves sciatica. The more supple you become the nearer you will be able to draw your leg down to your head.

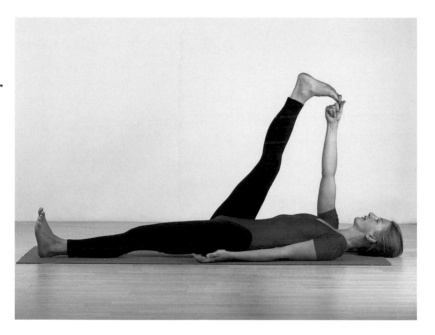

BENEFITS

- Stimulates the muscles of the legs.
- Helpful for low backache.
- Improves circulation in the lower half of the body.
- Tones the inner organs and the abdomen muscles.
- Helpful for flatulence.
- Stretches the hamstrings.

WATCH OUT!

- Approach with care if you have back problems.
- Take care if you have very tight hamstrings.

▼ Step 1

Lie with the back of your body flat on the floor,
your body in a straight line facing the ceiling.
Relax your arms by your sides; your palms
face upwards.

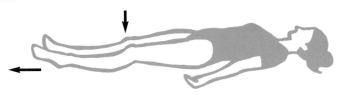

▲ Step 2

Bring your legs together, the inner-ankle bones,
knee joints and thighs touching. Push the backs
of your knees down into the floor, pull up with
the muscles and bones of your legs, and extend
your heels away from your body.

Step 3

Place your left palm on top of your left thigh,
fingers pointing to your toes. Push your lower
back down into the floor, and push your tailbone
down away from your waist.

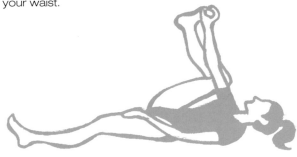

▲ Step 4

Breathe in; push your left thigh down with your
left hand, bend your right knee up towards your
chest. Bring your right arm to the inside of your
right leg and hook the index finger and thumb of
your right hand around your right big toe.

▼ Step 5

Breathe out; holding your right toe with your
right thumb and index finger, stretch your right
leg and arm up to the vertical. Straighten your
right leg, pushing the knee cap back and
pushing your heel away from your body.
Straighten your right arm, and lock your elbow.

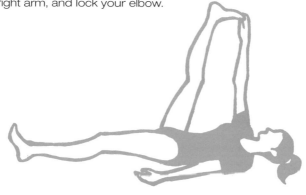

Step 6

Keep the back of your body and head firmly
down on the floor. Hold the posture and breathe
normally.

▼ Step 7

To come out of the posture: breathe out, release
your right big toe and lower your right leg down
onto the floor, in front of your body. Straighten
your legs. Lower your right arm down by your
side and relax both your arms by your sides,
palms facing the ceiling.

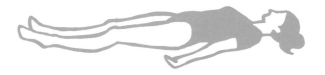

Step 8

Repeat the posture to the other side.

Salabhasana *Locust*

Salabhasana or Locust is a pose which requires strength. You may find that at first you are only able to raise your legs an inch or two off the ground, but it is worth persevering as this pose strengthens the lower back and tones the pelvic organs. The raising of the legs is achieved by pressing down onto your arms and the backs of your hands. Try to keep your shoulders soft throughout the pose and pull your shoulder blades together.

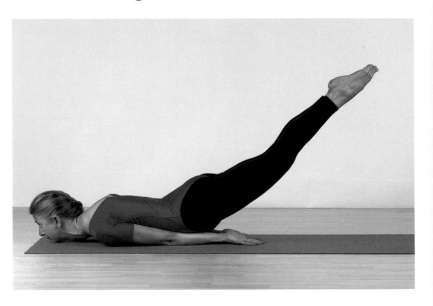

BENEFITS

- Strengthens legs and lower-back muscles.
- Firms the buttock muscles.
- Aids digestive problems.
- Flexes spine.

WATCH OUT!

- Avoid if you have abdominal problems.
- Take care if you have back problems.

▼ Step 1

Lie with your front on the floor and your body in a straight line. Rest one side of your head on the floor. Bring your legs and feet together; the tops of your feet rest on the floor, toes point back. Relax your arms by your sides; your palms face the ceiling.

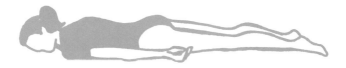

▼ Step 2

Put your chin on the floor, your face straight ahead. Slide your right arm and hand under your right side and your left arm and hand under your left side; your palms rest at the front of your thighs, fingers point down to your toes, and arms rest on the floor.

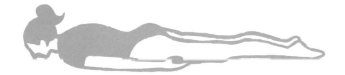

▼ Step 3

Breathe in; keep your chin on the floor. Push the backs of your arms and your hands into the floor and raise both your legs up behind your body; keep your pubic bone on the floor.

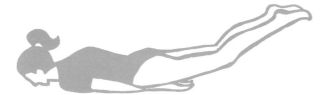

(continued)

▼ Step 4

Breathe out; bring your legs together and push your toes away from your body. Contract your buttock muscles, push your pubic bone and sacrum down to the floor and raise your legs as high as possible off the floor.

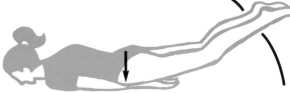

▲ Step 5

Rest your arms on the floor below your body, palms up. Hold the posture with your chin on floor; breathe normally.

▼ Step 6

Breathe out, lower your legs to the floor behind your body. Relax your arms by your sides, palms facing the ceiling. Rest your head on one side on the floor.

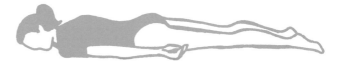

▼ Alternative Steps 3 & 4

If you cannot raise both legs off the floor behind your body, raise one at a time.

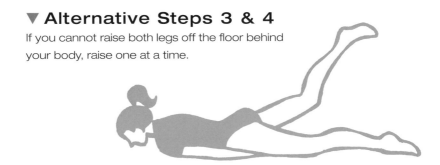

THE ASANAS

118

Dhanurasana *Bow*

Dhanurasana is a backbend. In this posture you rest on your abdomen, giving the digestive organs a good massage. Once you are comfortable in the pose, try rocking gently back and forth in time with your breathing. The kidneys are also massaged.

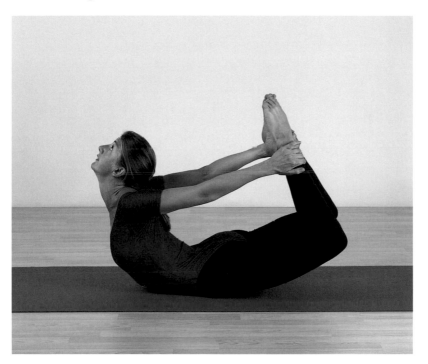

BENEFITS

- Expands the chest.
- Brings flexibility to the spine.
- Beneficial for slipped-disk problems.
- Relieves back pain.
- Tones arms and legs.
- Helps digestive problems.

WATCH OUT!

- Avoid if you have abdominal problems.
- Avoid if you have high blood pressure.
- Take care if you have knee, hip or back problems.

▼ Step 1

Lie with the front of your body on the floor and your body in a straight line. Rest one side of your head on the floor. Bring your legs and feet together; the tops of your feet rest on the floor, toes pointing back. Relax your arms by your sides.

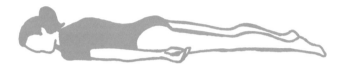

▼ Step 2

Place your chin on the floor. Bend your knees and bring the soles of your feet up behind your body towards your buttocks. Stretch your arms and hands back, and take hold of your right ankle with your right hand,and your left ankle with your left hand.

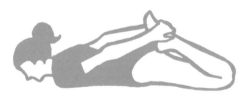

▼ Step 3

Breathe in; raise your chin off the floor and look straight ahead.

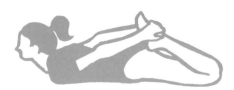

▼ Step 4

Breathe out; push the soles of your feet up towards the ceiling, away from your body. Pull your ankles up with your hands and raise your knees and thighs up off the floor (both legs lift evenly). At the same time, raise your head, shoulders and chest off the floor, and come up to balance on your abdomen.

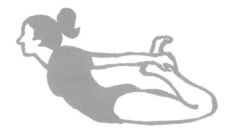

▼ Step 5

Bring your legs together with your inner ankles, knees and thighs touching. Take your shoulders back and push them down towards the floor, keeping them parallel. Slowly tilt your head back. Hold the posture, balancing on the abdomen and breathe normally.

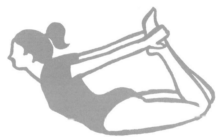

▼ Step 6

Release your ankles. Breathe out; lower your knees to the floor and extend your legs straight out onto the floor behind your body. Push your palms down into the floor and lower the front of your body to the floor. Relax your arms by your sides; your palms face the ceiling. Rest your head on one side. Relax the whole of the front of your body on the floor.

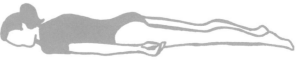

▶ Bhujangasana *Cobra*

As with all backward bends, the energy rises when you practise Bhujangasana. (In forward bends, the energy subsides.) In the final pose the navel must be barely off the ground. As well as working on the spine, keeping the bony structure flexible, it also keeps the spinal chord toned and refreshed. The compression on the lower body is good for keeping female reproductive organs healthy.

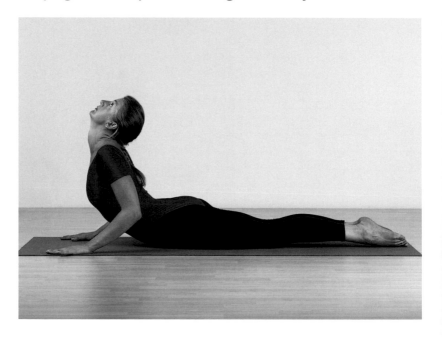

BENEFITS

- Helps respiratory problems.
- Strengthens the pectorals.
- Opens the chest.
- Beneficial for slipped-disk problems.
- Brings flexibility to the spine.
- Tones the buttocks.
- Aids digestion.

WATCH OUT!

- Be careful if you have back problems.
- Avoid if you have abdominal problems.
- Take care if you have arthritic wrists or shoulders.

▼ Step 1

Lie with the front of your body on the floor and your body in a straight line. Rest one side of your head on the floor. Bring your legs and feet together; the tops of your feet rest on the floor, toes pointing back. Relax your arms by sides, your palms facing the ceiling.

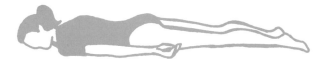

▼ Step 2

Place your forehead on the floor and the palms of your hands directly below your shoulders; your fingers spread wide and point forward. Bring your arms close to the sides of your body, your arms bent with elbows pointing towards your feet.

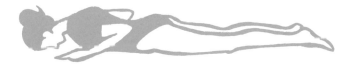

▼ Step 3

Breathe in; raise your head, shoulders and the front of your body up off the floor (keeping your pubic bone in contact with the floor).

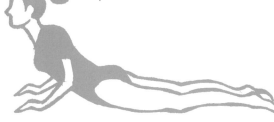

(continued)

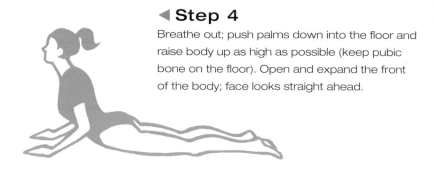

◀ Step 4

Breathe out; push palms down into the floor and raise body up as high as possible (keep pubic bone on the floor). Open and expand the front of the body; face looks straight ahead.

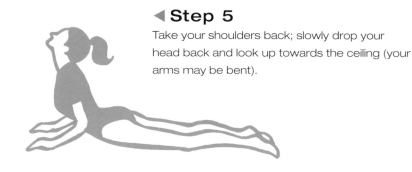

◀ Step 5

Take your shoulders back; slowly drop your head back and look up towards the ceiling (your arms may be bent).

Step 6

Relax your buttocks and leg muscles (feel your spine extending and flexing back). Hold the posture and breathe normally.

▼ Step 7

Push your palms into the floor. Breathe out; lower the front of your body down onto the floor. Rest one side of your head on the floor and relax your arms by the sides, your palms facing the ceiling. Relax the front of your body down into the floor.

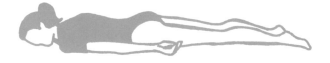

THE ASANAS

124

Urdhva mukha svanasana
Upward-facing dog

This is the natural counterpose to Adho mukha svanasana (Downward-facing dog). The only points of contact with the floor are the hands and backs of feet (or turned-in toes). The pelvis should be allowed to sink to the floor (but not touch it). This is a good pose for those suffering from a stiff back.

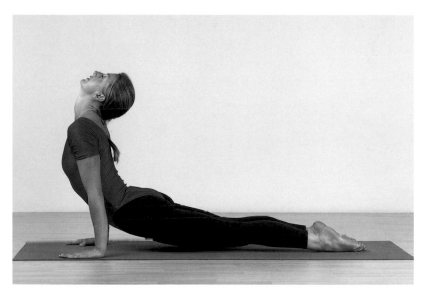

BENEFITS

- Strengthens and flexes the spine.
- Helps backache and pain.
- Beneficial for slipped-disk problems.
- Opens the front chest.
- Tones the pelvis and the abdomen.

WATCH OUT!

- Avoid if you have abdominal problems.
- Do not drop your head back if you have neck problems.
- Take care with eye and back problems.

▼ Step 1

Lie with the front of your body on the floor, your body in a straight line, legs together; the tops of your feet rest on the floor, toes pointing back. Rest one side of your head on the floor. Relax your arms by sides; the palms of your hands face the ceiling.

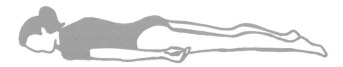

▼ Step 2

Place your chin on the floor. Take your feet 30 cm (1 ft) apart, toes pointing back. Bend your arms at the elbows and place the palms of your hands on the floor at either side of your chest, fingers pointing forward. Bring your arms close in beside your body; your elbows point down to the floor.

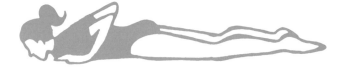

▶ Step 3

Breathe in; push the palms of your hands and the tops of your feet into the floor. Raise up your head, shoulders, body and thighs a little way off the floor.

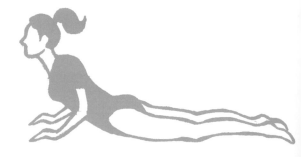

▼ Step 4

Breathe out; straighten your arms, pull your body and legs forward, bringing your chest through in front of your arms (your body curves back).

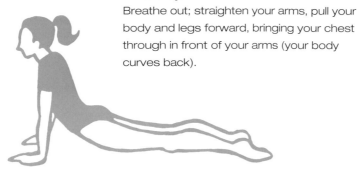

▼ Step 5

Roll your shoulders back and push them down towards your waist, keeping them parallel. Bring your shoulder blades closer together; relax your buttocks. Drop your head back and look up (feel the front of your body open and expand).

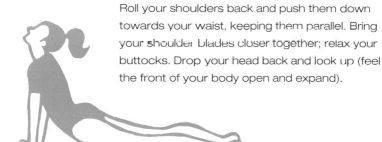

Step 6

Hold the posture, balancing your body weight on your palms and the tops of your feet, and breathe normally.

▼ Step 7

Breathe out; bend your arms and lower the front of your legs and body to the floor. Relax your head on one side, relax your arms by your sides, palms facing the ceiling.

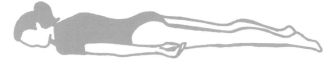

Bharadvajasana
Simple twist

Twists are wonderful for bringing fresh blood to the spine, keeping both the vertebrae and spinal cord toned. The simple twist works on the lumbar area. Always begin the twist from the lowest part of the spine and work it upwards. You can use the outbreath to relax further into the twist but take care not to lose height in the pose as you do so.

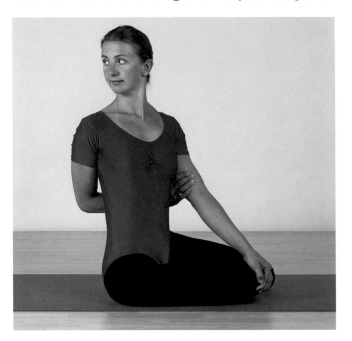

BENEFITS

- Strengthens and realigns the spine.
- Eases backache.
- Helps arthritis in the spine.
- Opens the chest.
- Tones the nervous system.

WATCH OUT!

- Take care if you have back or knee problems.
- Do not strain the back, neck or head.

▶ Step 1

Sit on both buttock bones, your spine straight, body facing forward and shoulders parallel. Bring your legs together, outstretched in front of your body. Relax your arms down by your sides. (See Dandasana, page 78.)

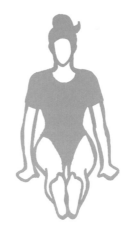

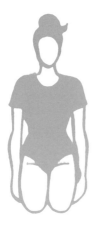

◀ Step 2

Bend your legs at the knees and bring your lower legs back by the side of your left buttock; your feet are beside your left buttock, knees pointing forward. Place your right foot under your left foot and rest your hands, palms down, on the floor beside hips.

▶ Step 3

Place your left hand, palm down, onto your right knee; your fingers remain relaxed. Place your right hand, palm down, onto the floor behind your body at base of your spine.

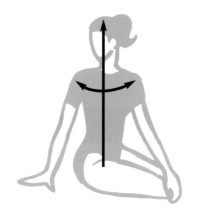

▲ Step 4

Breathe in; extend and stretch your spine upwards from your tailbone to the top of your head; open and expand the front of your body. Keep both buttocks on the floor.

(continued)

▼ Step 5

Breathe out; rotate your body from the hips round to the right. Rotate your whole spine and bring your left shoulder forward in line with your right shoulder.

▶ Step 6

Keeping your left arm straight, aim to take hold of your left upper arm with your right hand. Turn your head and look over the right shoulder.

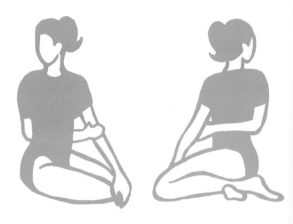

Step 7

Hold the posture, breathe normally. On each in-breath, stretch your body upwards, lifting and opening the chest; on each out-breath, rotate your body from the hips further round to the right, keeping your buttocks firmly on the floor.

▶ Step 8

Breathe in; rotate your body to the front, relax your arms by the sides. Breathe out; extend your legs straight out in front of your body.

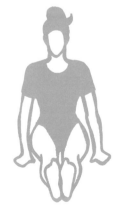

Step 9

Repeat the posture to the other side.

Maricyasana
Seated spinal twist

In this twist, if you cannot clasp your hands behind your back while keeping your spine straight, keep your left palm on the floor behind your body and put your right arm at the inside of your right knee. Bend your right arm, putting your elbow against the knee, right forearm vertical with palm facing your left leg and fingers pointing to the ceiling.

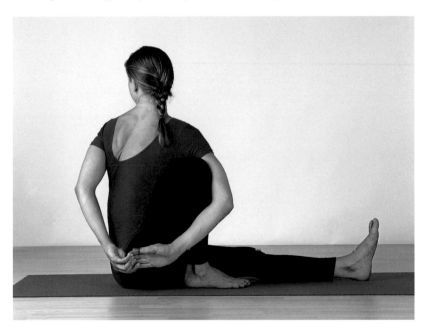

BENEFITS

- Opens the chest.
- Relaxes tight shoulders.
- Realigns the spine.
- Tones the abdomen.
- Beneficial for backache.
- Tones the nervous system.

WATCH OUT!

- Take care if you have abdominal problems.
- Approach with care if you have backache or back problems.

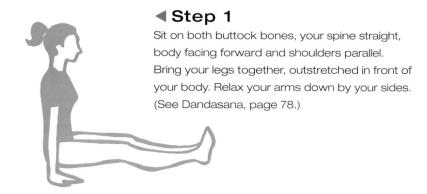

◀ Step 1

Sit on both buttock bones, your spine straight, body facing forward and shoulders parallel. Bring your legs together, outstretched in front of your body. Relax your arms down by your sides. (See Dandasana, page 78.)

▶ Step 2

Bend your right leg and bring your right heel close into your right thigh; your right knee points up to the ceiling. Extend your left leg straight out in front of your body, push your heel away from your body; your toes point up toward the ceiling.

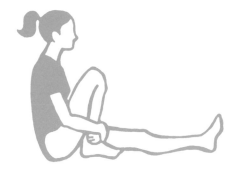

◀ Step 3

Stretch your spine upwards and turn your body from the hips, to the left. Take your left arm back behind your body and place your left palm down onto the floor at base of your spine, your fingers pointing back and your left arm straight.

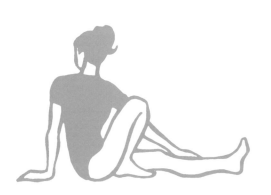

THE ASANAS

132

▶ Step 4

Bring your right arm to the inside of your right leg and take it around the leg (from the inside to the outside), and bring your right hand behind your back. Raise your left hand off the floor and clasp hands together behind your back.

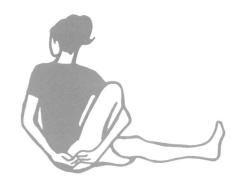

Step 5

Breathe in; extend and stretch your spine upwards from the tailbone to the top of your head; open and expand the front of your body.

◀ Step 6

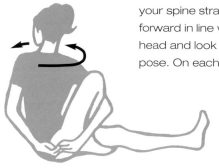

Breathe out; rotate your body from the hips round to the left, rotating all of your spine. Keep your spine straight and bring your right shoulder forward in line with your left shoulder; turn your head and look over your left shoulder. Hold the pose. On each in-breath extend and stretch your body up; on each out-breath, twist your body further to the left, rotating at the hips; keep both buttocks on the floor.

◀ Step 7

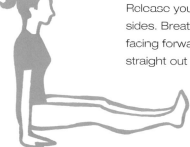

Release your hands and relax your arms by your sides. Breathe in; rotate your body to the front, facing forward. Breathe out; extend your legs straight out in front of your body.

Step 8

Repeat the pose to the other side.

Jathara parivatanasana
Lying twist

In this twist, if you cannot stretch both your legs straight up to the vertical, bend your knees and bring them close to the chest, and take your legs down onto the floor at the sides of your body – with your legs bent. See page 137.

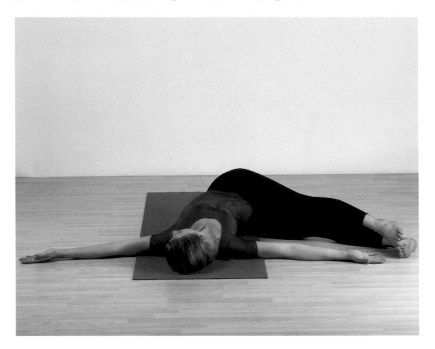

BENEFITS

- Stimulates and tones the abdominal organs.
- Strengthens the intestines.
- Helps reduce flab around the area of the waist and hips.
- Helps gastric problems.
- Eases lower-back and hip pain.

WATCH OUT!

- Do not do if you have arthritis in the hips.
- Do not raise legs to the vertical if you have abdominal or lower-back problems.

THE ASANAS

▼ Step 1

Lie flat on your back, your body in a straight line; your shoulders and hips are parallel. Relax your arms by your sides.

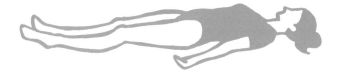

▼ Step 2

Extend your arms out by your sides at shoulder level; your palms face the ceiling.

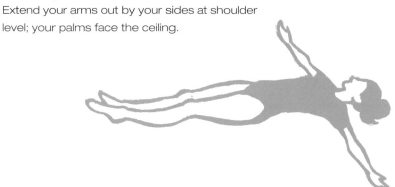

▶ Step 3

Breathe in; raise both your legs straight up to the vertical (you can do this by bending your knees over your stomach and then straightening them. Push your heels towards the ceiling and flatten the soles of your feet; your toes point in towards your face.

(continued)

▼ Step 4

Breathe out; rotate at your right hip and slowly
lower your legs straight down towards the floor
at the right side of your body. If your feet touch
the floor, slide your toes up towards your right
hand and push your heels away from your body
to stretch out the backs of your legs.

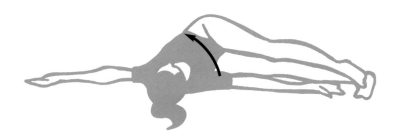

Step 5

Roll your abdomen and stomach to the left and
relax the back of your body; keep your left hip,
ribcage and left shoulder down on the floor.

▼ Step 6

Keep both your shoulders on the floor, shoulders
parallel. Relax your neck and head and slowly
turn your head to the left and look towards your
left hand. Hold the posture; breathe normally.

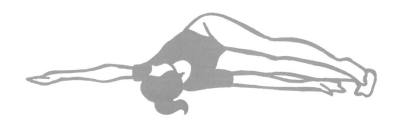

▶ Step 7

Push the backs of your arms and hands into the floor and breathe in; raise your legs to the vertical and breathe out.

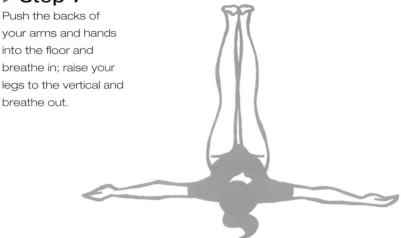

Step 8

Repeat posture to the other side from Step 3.

▼ Alternative Steps 3–6

If you cannot raise your legs in the air, bend your knees to bring your legs close to your chest and lower them, still bent, and twist.

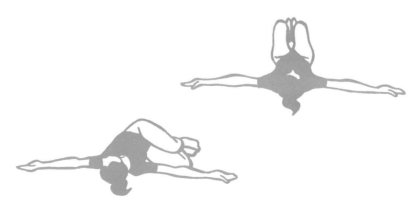

▶ Ardha navasana *Boat*

Ardha navasana is a balance posture. If your breathing becomes strained in the pose, breathe towards your upper chest. Keep your abdominal muscles relaxed, and do not let the base of your spine come onto the floor.

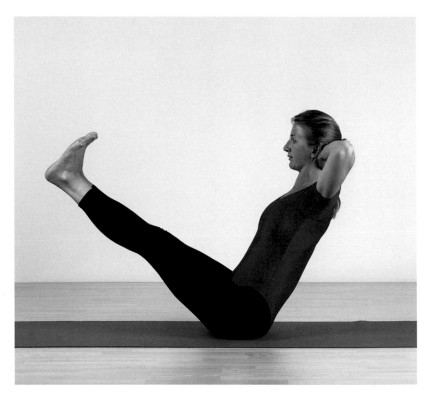

BENEFITS

- Strengthens the back muscles.
- Tones and stimulates the abdominal organs.
- Helps to trim the waist.
- Tones the kidneys, improving their function.

WATCH OUT!

- Do not do in the early stages of pregnancy.
- Take care if you have abdominal or back problems.

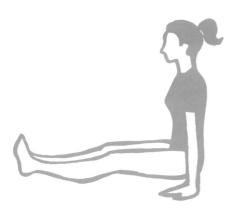

◀ Step 1

Sit on both buttock bones, your spine straight, body facing forward and shoulders parallel. Bring your legs together, outstretched in front of your body. Relax your arms down by your sides. (See Dandasana, page 78.)

▶ Step 2

Interlink your fingers and place your palms on the base of your head. Extend your elbows out to the sides.

▶ Step 3

Breathe in, and stretch your spine upwards from the tailbone to the top of your head. Open and stretch front of your body.

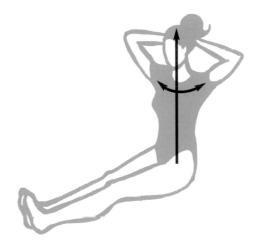

◀ Step 4

Breathe out; lean your body back from base to a 30° angle and raise both legs straight out in front of your body to a 30° angle (your buttock bones remain on the floor).

(continued)

▶ Step 5

Push your heels away from your body, push back your kneecaps and pull up with the leg muscles and bones; point your toes in to the forehead (aim to bring your toes in line with top of head). Hold the posture, balanced, and breathe normally.

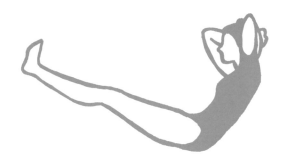

Step 6

Hold the posture, balanced, and breathe normally.

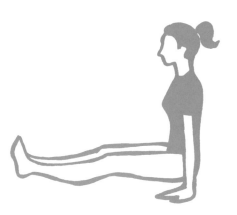

◀ Step 7

Breathe out; lower your legs to the floor in front of your body. Straighten your body to the vertical, release your hands and relax your arms. Place your hands down by your sides.

Paripurna navasana
Boat with oars

Paripurna navasana is a balance posture and throughout you should aim to keep lifting the body and opening the front chest. If your breathing becomes strained, breathe towards your upper chest. Keep your abdominal muscles relaxed, and do not let the base of your spine come onto the floor.

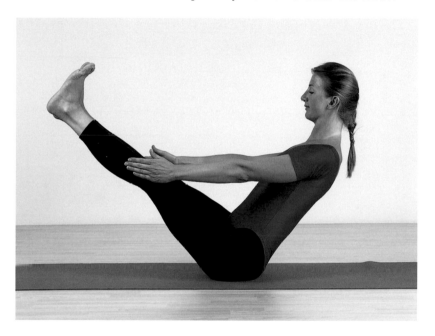

BENEFITS

- Strengthens the back muscles.
- Tones and stimulates the abdominal organs.
- Helps to trim the waist.
- Tones the kidneys, improving their function.
- Aids a bloated abdomen and gastric problems.

WATCH OUT!

- Do not do in early pregnancy.
- Take care if you have abdominal or back problems.
- Avoid if you have high blood pressure.

▶ Step 1

Sit on both buttock bones, your spine straight,
body facing forward and shoulders parallel.
Bring your legs together, outstretched in front of
your body. Relax your arms down by your sides.
(See Dandasana, page 78.)

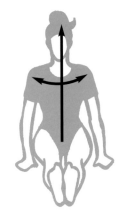

◀ Step 2

Breathe in; stretch your spine upwards from the
tailbone to the top of your head. Open and
stretch up the front of your body.

▼ Step 3

Breathe out; lean your body backwards from the
base to a 60° degree angle and raise both your
legs straight up in front to a 60° degree angle.
Your toes point towards forehead and your heels
push away (your feet are
higher than the head).
Your buttock bones
remain on the floor.

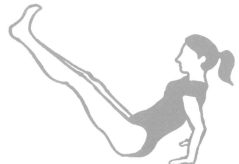

▶ Step 4

Extend your arms straight out in front of your body keeping them in line with your shoulders. Bring your palms to the outside of your knees; your palms face each other, and fingers point forward.

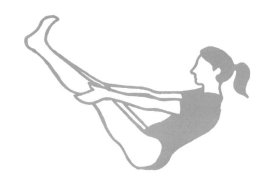

Step 5

Hold the posture, balancing on your buttock bones, and breathe normally.

▶ Step 6

Breathe out; lower your legs to the floor, straighten your body to the vertical and lower your arms to your sides.

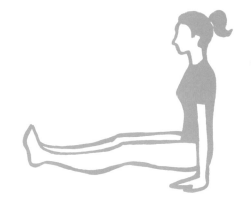

Adho mukha svanasana
Downward-facing dog

This is one of the 'easier' upside-down poses where your heart is higher than your head and the blood flows down into the upper chest and head. This brings fresh blood to the brain and the important glands located there and in the upper chest: thyroid, pineal and pituitary. It is also a refreshing pose which restores energy.

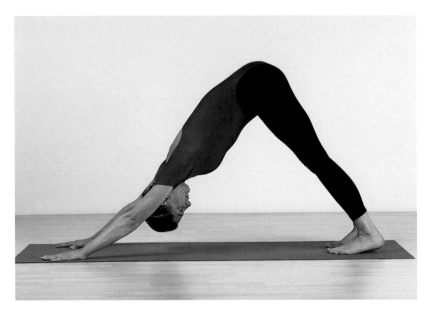

THE ASANAS

144

BENEFITS

- Stimulates the body.
- Strengthens leg and arm joints.
- Stretches the spine.
- Relieves tiredness.
- Loosens the hips and shoulders.
- Increases circulation.

WATCH OUT!

- Take care if you have arthritic wrists.
- Do not do if you have eye problems.
- Avoid if you have abnormal blood pressure.

▶ Step 1

From a kneeling position, come up onto your hands and knees.

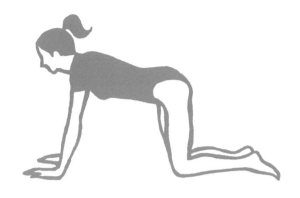

◀ Step 2

Place your hands, palms down, directly below your shoulders, shoulder-width apart; your fingers point forward. Place your knees directly below your hips, hip-width apart. Tuck your toes under; your heels point up towards the ceiling.

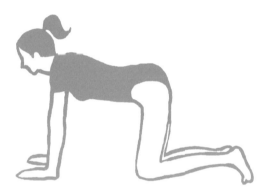

▶ Step 3

Walk your palms 15 cm (6 in) forward, still shoulder-width apart. Keeping your palms and toes on the floor, breathe out; push your hips and tailbone up towards the ceiling. Push your heels down towards the floor (feel your legs stretch out and strengthen).

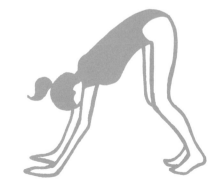

(continued)

▶ Step 4

Stretch your arms out
fully in front of your
body, shoulder-width
apart. Press the heels
of your hands into the
floor, squeeze your
shoulder blades
together and push
your shoulders down
towards your waist.

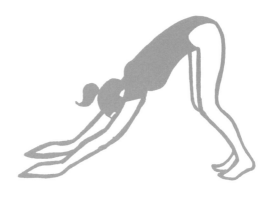

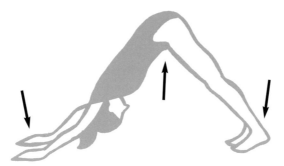

◀ Step 5

Drop your head and
body down through
your arms; the top of
the head faces the
floor. Relax your head
and neck.

▲ Step 6

Push your hands and heels down into the floor,
push your tailbone up towards the ceiling and
spread your buttocks wide (the body's weight is
evenly distributed between hands and feet).
Hold the posture and breathe normally.

▶ Step 7

To come out: walk your hands in towards your
feet. Bend your knees and place them on the
floor; your shins and the tops of feet rest on the
floor, toes pointing back. Place your buttocks
onto your heels, straighten your body up; your
body faces forward. Relax your arms by your
sides.

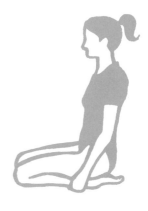

Halasana *Plough*

Halasana, or the Plough, is a classic inverted posture. If you find it too hard to take your toes down onto the floor behind your head, put them instead onto a chair or, if you can manage, onto one or two folded blankets. The chin pressed into the chest massages the thyroid gland which regulates the body's metabolism.

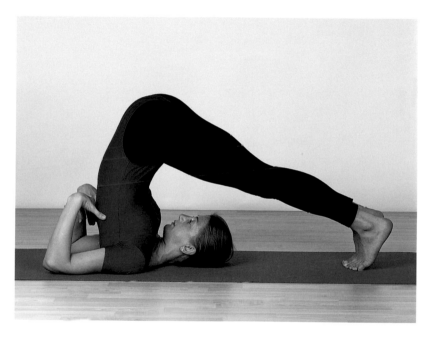

BENEFITS

- Aids digestive disorders and high blood pressure.
- Flexes the spine.
- Stimulates the abdominal organs.
- Tones the nervous system.
- Improves circulation and re-energizes the body.
- Stimulates the thyroid gland.

WATCH OUT!

- Do not practise if you have hip, lower-back, neck, shoulder or blood-pressure problems.
- Take care doing this pose during your period.

▼ Step 1

Lie flat on your back, your body in a straight line. Relax your arms your sides, your palms on the floor.

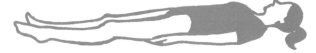

◀ Step 2

Breathe in; bend your knees up onto your chest, push your palms down into the floor and raise your buttocks and hips off the floor to bring your knees towards your forehead.

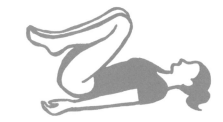

◀ Step 3

Place your palms onto your back, supporting your body, and straighten up your spine (bring your elbows into line with your shoulders).

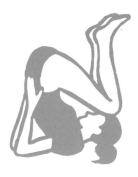

▶ Step 4

Breathe out; extend your legs out over past your face and bring your toes down onto the floor; tuck your toes under towards your head.

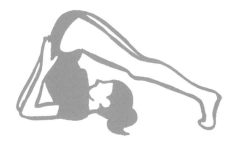

Step 5

Keeping your toes on the floor, lift your ankles, shins, knees and thighs and push them up towards the ceiling. Push your heels away from your body, straightening your legs.

THE ASANAS

148

▶ Step 6

Turn your hands
so that your fingers
point down. Push your
buttock bones up
towards the ceiling,
straightening and
stretching your spine

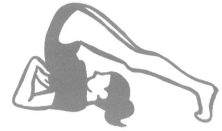

and spreading your buttocks wide. Hold the
posture and breathe normally.

▼ Step 7

To come out: breathe out, bring your arms
down onto the floor in front of your body,
keeping them straight in line with your
shoulders. Push your palms and arms down into
the floor and, keeping the back of your head on
the floor, slowly uncurl your spine down onto the
floor. Bring your legs to the vertical and lower
them down in front of your body to the floor
(your legs can be bent). Relax the back of your
body to the floor and
relax your arms by
your sides, your legs
outstretched in front
of the body.

Advanced pose

If you can take the posture further, bring your
arms and hands down onto the floor in front of
your body. Interlink your fingers and push your
palms away from your body, with the outside
edges of your hands and little fingers resting on
the floor. Straighten your arms, lock out your
elbows and push your arms down into the floor.
Stretch your spine up to the ceiling.

▶ Setu bandha *Bridge*

Setu bandha, or Bridge, opens the chest, realigns the spine and cures round shoulders. The stretch over the stomach means that the digestive organs are toned. It can also help relieve menstrual problems.

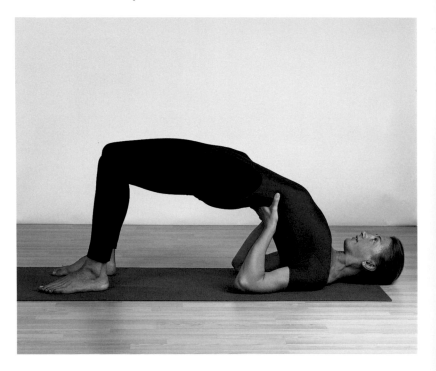

BENEFITS

- Helps respiratory problems.
- Opens the front of the body.
- Flexes the spine.
- Tones the nervous system.
- Strengthens the legs.
- Tones the hips and thighs.

WATCH OUT!

- Do not practise if you have severe abdominal problems.
- Take care if you have back or knee problems.
- Avoid if you have stiff or arthritic hips.

▼ Step 1

Lie with your back flat on the floor and your body in a straight line. Relax your arms by sides, palms up.

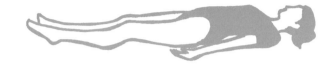

◀ Step 2

Bend your knees and place the soles of your feet flat on the floor. Bring your heels close in towards your buttocks, the feet parallel and hip-width apart; your toes point forward and knees point up towards the ceiling.

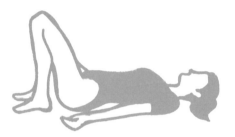

▼ Step 3

Breathe in; raise your buttocks and the back of your body up off the floor. Push the soles of your feet into the floor, tighten the buttock and thigh muscles and push your pelvis, hips and the front of your body up towards the ceiling. Your body lifts upwards to rest on the shoulders.

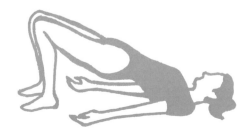

(continued)

▼ Step 4

Breathe out; place your arms below your body, bend your elbows and place your palms onto the back of your waist; your upper arms stay in contact with the floor. Walk your heels (hip-width apart) closer in towards your shoulders and push your pelvis, hips and the front of your body further up towards the ceiling, extending and pushing your knees forwards towards your feet (knees hip-width apart).

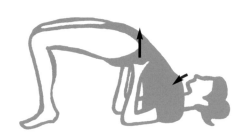

▲ Step 5

Relax your shoulders and the back of your head on the floor. Tuck your chin in towards your chest to lengthen the back of your neck (feel your body lift upwards and curve back). Hold the posture and breathe normally, balancing your body weight on the soles of your feet, shoulders and the back of your head. (A variation is to come up on your toes.)

▼ Step 6

Breathe out; bring your arms down by your sides, palms down. Push your palms and arms into the floor and slowly uncurl your spine from top to bottom down onto the floor. Relax your back on the floor, stretch your legs straight out in front of your body and relax your arms by your sides.

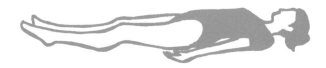

Viparita karani
Legs up wall

Viparita karani is a restful, inverted posture which is good for people who spend much of the day on their feet. Try breathing out through the back of the waist and you will feel your lower back relaxing onto the floor.

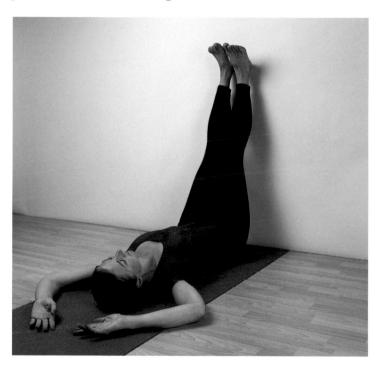

BENEFITS

- Improves lower-body circulation.
- Opens the front of the body.
- Rejuvenates tired legs.
- Releases lower-back tension.
- Relaxes the entire body.

WATCH OUT!

- Do not take arms over head if you have blood-pressure or heart problems.
- Take care if you have hip problems.

▼ Step 1

Lie, your back on floor, legs outstretched and heels resting on a wall. Relax your arms by sides, palms up.

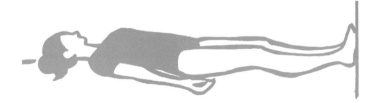

Step 2

Bend your knees to your chest; bring your buttocks in towards the wall.

◀ Step 3

With your knees bent, place the soles of your feet on the wall, hip-width apart.

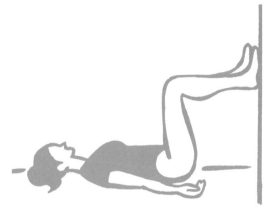

▶ Step 4

Bring your buttocks in as close to the wall as is comfortable and extend your legs straight up, together. Push your heels up; your toes point towards your head (your back rests on the floor).

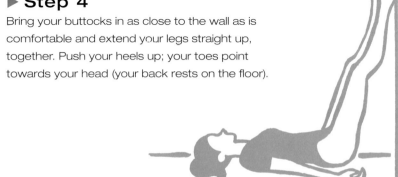

THE ASANAS

154

▶ Step 5

Take your arms over past your head, arms slightly bent, and relax them onto the floor; your palms face the ceiling.

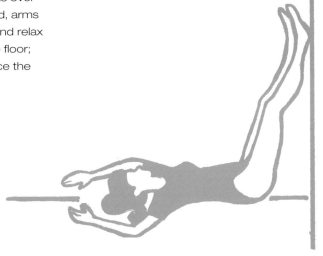

Step 6

Relax the back of your body down onto the floor, ensuring your hips and shoulders are parallel; your legs rest in a vertical position up against the wall.

Step 7

Hold the posture and breathe normally.

▼ Step 8

Bring your arms forward by your sides. Push your body back from the wall, and bring your legs down to the floor and straighten them. Relax your back.

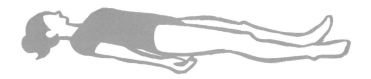

how to

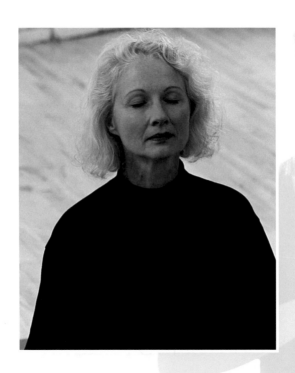

relax

Relaxation is an important element of yoga. Its purpose is to bring stillness to the body and mind and eliminate outside thoughts, so letting you concentrate – the first step to meditation. The art of relaxation is also a very useful skill to learn: once mastered, it can be applied at other times in your daily life. This chapter will introduce you to some basic relaxation techniques.

The relaxation session

A relaxation session should always come at the end of a class or your own personal yoga practice. Ideally, it should last for at least 10 minutes (but this also depends on the length of the yoga session; see p. 176).

Practical considerations

Before beginning any relaxation session, bear in mind the following guidelines.

The room should be at a comfortable temperature. The body cools down very quickly when lying still and if you begin to feel cool you will be unable to relax, so make sure you have a jumper and socks to put on or a blanket to cover yourself.

Minimize distractions like TV, traffic or music. Half-draw the curtains to darken the room and make sure no-one will disturb you.

BENEFITS

- Refreshes mind and body.
- Invigorates nerve cells.
- Increases creativity.
- Promotes a calm, clear mind.
- Lowers blood pressure.
- Increases blood supply to vital organs.

BASIC RELAXATION

- Lie in Corpse (see p. 102).
- Make sure your body is in line: head, chest, hips and ankles.
- Feet should be a few inches apart, falling outwards.
- Arms lie alongside the body, hands a few inches from the hips. Palms face the ceiling (this opens the chest), fingers gently curled.
- Neck should be long with the chin slightly tucked in. If it doesn't feel long, lift your head up slightly, then lay it down vertebra by vertebra. Alternatively, place a small pillow below the nape of your neck.

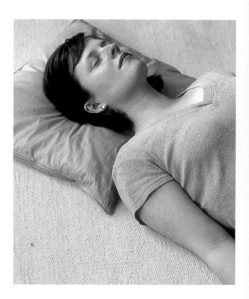

▲ If your neck is tense or strained, support it and your head with a small pillow.

Tension points

Now that you are in the correct position, try to be aware of any tension points in your body.

Lower back

Is your lower back tense? Is there a large gap between your lower back and the ground? As much as possible of your spine should touch the ground. Slip your hand under the small of your back then try to relax so your back sinks down onto your hand.

Alternatively, place a cushion beneath your knees; this will help to lower your back onto the floor.

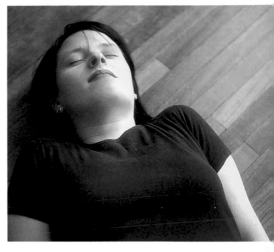

▲ It is important not to let neck muscles contract and scrunch up.

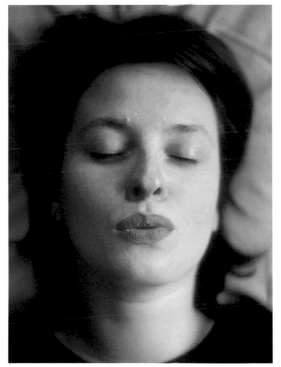

▲ Are your mouth and jaws clenched? It's easy to keep your face muscles tense without realizing it.

Shoulders

Are your shoulders creeping up to meet your ears? Shoulders should be wide and relaxed and your neck should be long. If you need to, place a small cushion beneath the nape of the neck.

Face

Is there tension in your face? Lips should be slightly parted, your tongue should even be relaxed. Eyes should be shut with the eyeballs soft beneath the relaxed lids. Try to feel as though your face is smiling softly.

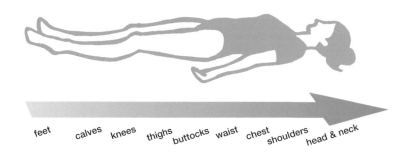

feet   calves   knees   thighs   buttocks   waist   chest   shoulders   head & neck

Body scanning

Once you feel comfortable and relaxed, release the tension from your muscles using the body scanning technique. Focus your attention on each body part in turn, beginning with your feet and gradually moving up to your head.

Feet: the skin on the soles, each one of your toes, insteps, ankles. Feel them relax, grow soft and gentle.

Legs: calves, knees, thighs. Feel them relax, grow soft and gentle and heavy. Let the ground take the weight of your legs.

Hips, buttocks and the muscles at the base of the spine: feel them relax, grow soft and gentle.

Waist, tummy, sides, ribcage, upper back: feel them relax, grow soft and gentle.

Shoulders: focus on the right shoulder and move down the right arm: top, elbow, forearm, wrist, palm of the hand, each finger in turn. Feel them relax, grow soft and gentle. Now switch your focus to the left shoulder and as before, move down the arm: top, elbow, forearm, wrist, palm of the hand, each finger in turn. Feel them relax, grow soft and gentle.

Neck and throat: feel them relax, grow soft and gentle.

Face: chin, lower jaw, mouth (let the lips part slightly), tongue, cheeks, nose. Feel them relax, grow soft and gentle.

Eyes: eyelids should be gently closed over the eyeballs, the eyeballs should be soft.

MUST KNOW

Breathing
Breathing should be through the nostrils, slow, steady, rhythmic. As you lie on the ground, become aware of your breath. Don't force it, just observe how it is coming and going. Watch how your tummy rises and falls in a slow, regular rhythm.

Forehead, scalp and ears: there should be no frown lines. Your face is completely soft. Feel them relax, grow soft and gentle. Your head should be heavy on the floor. Your whole body should be fully relaxed.

As you become completely relaxed, you will feel the pull of gravity. Your body will feel heavier and heavier and you will let the ground take all the weight. You may not feel this the first time, but as you continue practising you will begin to recognize the feeling of total relaxation and it will be easier to achieve.

The mind during relaxation

At first it is hard not to let thoughts intrude. But tell yourself the relaxation session is a time to let your mind have a rest, too – it needs a chance to be completely blank. If you find thoughts flitting into your mind, push them gently aside, taking no notice of them. Gradually you feel divorced from your body as though you are floating outside it. It is as though you can observe yourself lying on the mat.

Coming out of relaxation

When the session is over, take your awareness back to your body lying on the ground. Muscles and nerves have to be reawakened and brought back to the present. Do this by slowly moving fingers and toes, clenching and unclenching them. Then begin to stretch the body – hands and fingers stretch upwards along the ground, heels push downwards. As you stretch, let yourself yawn fully as though waking from a deep sleep. Stretch and yawn.

To come up to a sitting position from Corpse, turn onto your right side and slowly push yourself up into a sitting position, taking care to let your head come up slowly. Keep your eyes looking down. Once up, slowly open your eyes.

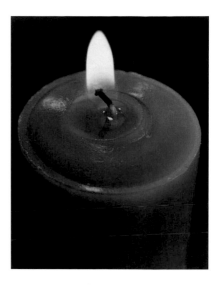

▲ When relaxing, focus your attention on an inanimate object, such as a candle, to prevent your mind from wandering.

want to know more?

Take it to the next level...

Go to...
▶ **Head and neck exercises** – page 32
▶ **Breathing exercises** – page 166
▶ **Home sessions** – page 176

Other sources
▶ **Qualified yoga teacher**
  for relaxation tips and advice
▶ **Retreats**
  for relaxation and meditation breaks
▶ **Magazines**
  for relaxation features
▶ **Internet**
  for meditation and relaxation sites
▶ **Publications**
  visit www.thorsons.com for books on yoga

yogic

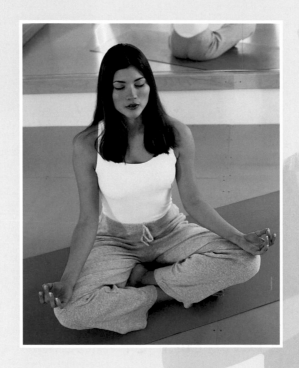

breath

Yogic breathing or *pranayama* is recognized as one of the main ways to refresh and rejuvenate all the body systems. *Prana* has several meanings: breath, respiration, life, vitality, wind, energy and strength, while *yama* is restraint or discipline. In this chapter, we'll explore the ways the body channels *prana* energy and exercises to help control it.

163

Energy flow

Just as blood circulates through a network of veins and arteries, *prana* is believed to flow through the body along an extensive network of channels known as *nadi*. The main channel and most important *nadi* runs along the spinal column and is known as *sushumna*.

The chakras

Situated along the line of the spine are seven major energy centres known as *chakras* (from the Sanskrit, meaning 'wheel'), with a further 122 minor ones situated in our joints, bones and nerves. The illustration below shows each of the major chakras and their locations.

Energy flows within the body from the crown *chakra* (*Sahasrara*) down along the line of the spine through all the other major energy centres. It is important to keep this main energy channel clear with the 'wheels' turning smoothly since blockages of the energy flow between them can cause physical and mental problems. For example, a blockage in the *Manipura chakra* (in the navel area) can result in anger and digestive disorders while

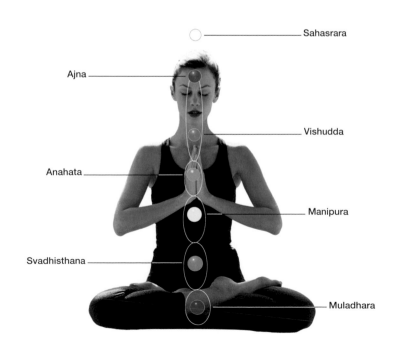

Sahasrara

Ajna

Vishudda

Anahata

Manipura

Svadhisthana

Muladhara

a blockage in the *Anahata chakra*, also known as the heart centre, might result in difficulty in expressing emotion.

In yoga, the breath is used to direct the flow of prana through the body, avoiding blockages and rejuvenating all the body systems.

THE CHAKRAS

Sahasrara chakra
Location: crown of head
Influences: pineal gland   *Colour*: white (or violet)
Represents: enlightenment, bliss   *Mantra*: om (long)

Ajna chakra
Location: middle of forehead (third eye)
Influences: pituitary gland, nervous system   *Colour*: indigo
Represents: intuition, wisdom   *Mantra*: om (short)

Vishudda chakra
Location: throat
Influences: thyroid gland, throat, lungs   *Colour*: blue
Represents: higher knowledge, learning   *Mantra*: ham

Anahata chakra
Location: centre of chest (heart centre)
Influences: heart and blood circulation   *Colour*: green
Represents: love, compassion, emotions   *Mantra*: yam

Manipura chakra
Location: navel (solar plexus)
Influences: digestive system   *Colour*: yellow
Represents: willpower, self assertion   *Mantra*: ram

Svadhisthana chakra
Location: genital area
Influences: reproduction, growth   *Colour*: orange
Represents: growth, preservation   *Mantra*: vam

Muladhara chakra
Location: base of spine (anus)
Influences: elimination processes   *Colour*: red
Represents: physical strength, stability   *Mantra*: lam

▶ Breathing exercises

The exercises that follow show the main yogic breathing techniques. It is always best to do these initially under the supervision of a qualified yoga teacher.

> **WATCH OUT!**
>
> **Pranayama**
> Pranayama is a powerful technique and care should be taken when practising. If you feel your breathing becoming uncomfortable or you feel dizzy, stop immediately, lie down and relax. If it makes you feel over-emotional you should stop.

Learning to breathe

Most people use only the top portion of their lungs to breathe, taking only shallow breaths. Full yogic breathing involves all the lungs – the top part beneath the collarbones and shoulders, the middle part beneath the ribcage and the bottom part (the largest area) above the diaphragm.

Breathing and the chakras

By focusing on each of the chakras in turn and then 'breathing into' them using the exercises, you can boost the flow of energy.

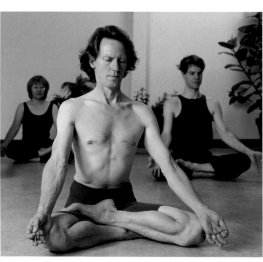

> **MUST KNOW**
>
> **Spine straight**
> When you practise breathing, it is essential that you keep your spine erect for the energy to travel freely along its length.

◀ If you are not taught these exercises in class, ask your teacher for advice and guidance.

YOGIC BREATH

166

- Calms and quietens the mind.
- Strengthens the immune system.
- Improves concentration.
- Increases the capacity of the lungs.
- Refreshes both the body and mind.
- Improves circulation of the blood.

Eating and breathing
If you are planning to practise yogic breathing, then wait at least two hours after your last meal. Also, do not practise if you're hungry.

Beginning with the crown chakra, visualize the corresponding colour as you do this and focus on the body locations and influences governed by each chakra in turn. Sounding the mantra that relates to each also increases the flow of energy through each chakra.

Complete breath

Posture: seated or lying down.

Step 1
Start by expelling the air from your lungs by pulling in the stomach muscles gently. Release the squeeze and begin to inhale deeply, taking the air into the lowest portion of your lungs.

Step 2
Feel the air filling the middle portion of the lungs and then the top potion of your lungs. You may feel some movement across your shoulders.

Step 3
Exhale slowly and fully begin expelling the air from the top of the lungs, then the middle and finally the bottom part of the lungs. Pull in the tummy muscles gently to squeeze any air left in the bottom of the lungs. Relax the squeeze.

Continue for as long as you like.

- Increases oxygen levels in blood.
- Tones the nervous system.

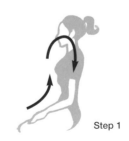

Step 1

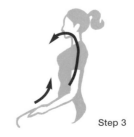

Step 3

YOGIC BREATH

167

Cleansing breath (*Ha* breath)

Posture: seated or standing. Here, it is described in a standing position.

Step 1

Stand with feet hip-width apart. Clasp hands together, arms straight.

Step 2

Inhale fully as you take your arms up above your head.

Step 3

Exhale through the mouth with a 'ha' sound as you bend forward at the waist. Arms swing through the legs; bend your knees slightly at the same time and pull in abdominal muscles to squeeze out all air from the bottom of the lungs; remain in the position without inhaling.

Step 4

Exhale again through the mouth with a sigh to get rid of any further stale air in the lungs.

Step 5

Inhale deeply as you straighten up with knees slightly bent. Arms come up above your head.

Repeat three times.

WATCH OUT!

Cleansing breath
- Do not do if you have high blood pressure, eye problems or a hiatus hernia.
- Stop if you feel dizzy or hyperventilate.

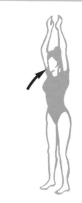

Step 2

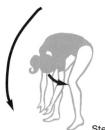

Step 3

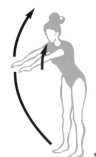

Step 5

Alternate nostril breathing (*Nadi sodana*)

Posture: seated.

Step 1
Sit comfortably with your spine straight. Begin by breathing slowly and regularly so that you become relaxed.

Step 2
Take your right hand and fold the index and middle finger into your palm. The thumb, fourth and little fingers are straight.

Step 3
Close the right nostril with the thumb and inhale fully and slowly through the left nostril. (Some schools of yoga keep the index and middle fingers straight, resting gently on the forehead between the eyes, while using the thumb and little fingers to close each of the nostrils.

Step 4
Close the left nostril with the fourth and little fingers and exhale through the right. Pause and then inhale through the same nostril (the right).

Step 5
Close the right nostril and exhale through the left.

This completes one cycle. Start again inhaling through the left nostril and complete three cycles.

BENEFITS
- Lowers stress levels.
- Calms the mind.
- Aids good sleep.
- Helps develop concentration.

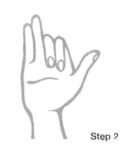

Step 2

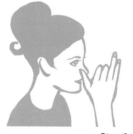

Step 3

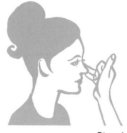

Step 4

YOGIC BREATH

Victorious breath (*Ujjayi* breath)

- Strengthens nervous system.
- Aids circulation.
- Improves lung tissue.
- Quietens the mind.

Posture: Easy Pose (p. 85) or Hero (p. 80).

Step 1

Let your head fall forward onto your chest so your chin is pressed into your breastbone.

Step 2

Stretch out your arms and rest the back of your hands on your knees. Join the tips of the index fingers and thumbs, leaving other fingers straight (this hand gesture is known as *hasta mudra*). Exhale fully.

Step 3

Inhale slowly and steadily through the nostrils. As the air is drawn in there is a hissing sound (sa) caused by the chin lock. Fill the lungs and pause.

Step 4

Exhale slowly and steadily. The air brushing past the palate will again make a sound (ha). Once the lungs are empty, pause.

Repeat for a few minutes with eyes closed. Focus on the two different sounds.

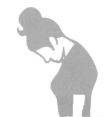

Step 1

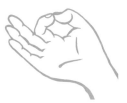

Step 2

WATCH OUT!

Victorious breath
- Do not do if you have heart or lung problems.

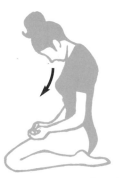

Step 4

Bellows breath
(*Bhastrika*)

Note: this should only be learned under the guidance of an experienced yoga teacher.

Posture: seated.

Step 1
Inhale smoothly and deeply.

Step 2
Exhale forcefully, using your abdominal muscles to push out the air through your nostrils. Feel as though you are trying to push something out of your nose.

Step 3
Immediately breathe in using the same force – your abdomen is pushed out.

Step 4
Repeat the forced exhalation with the inhalation following. Picture bellows stoking a fire. Your abdomen moves in and out with the same force.

Practise initially for about 10 seconds. Once you master the technique you will be able to continue for longer.

BENEFITS

● Highly cleansing and rids body toxins.
● Good for circulation.
● Good for sinuses.
● Clears mind and aids concentration.
● Tones digestive organs.
● Strengthens nervous system.

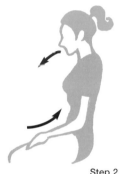

Step 2

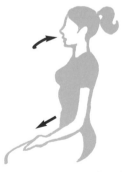

Step 3

YOGIC BREATH

171

Cooling breath (*Sitali*)

BENEFITS

- Relaxes the nervous system.
- Soothes eyes, ears.
- Cooling.
- Good for digestion and liver.

Note: being able to curl your tongue – essential for this exercise – is a genetic trait which you either have or you don't. It can't be learned so if you can't curl your tongue, you never will.

Posture: seated with hands resting on knees (in *hasta mudra* if preferred – see p. 170).

Step 1
Begin by breathing regularly slowly and smoothly to relax your body.

Step 2
Stick your tongue out as far as you can. Curl up the sides of your tongue into a tube.

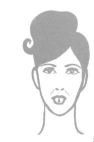

Step 2

Step 3
Inhale slowly, drawing the air through the tube made by your tongue. The air feels cool against your tongue and also on the roof of your mouth.

Step 4
At the end of the in-breath, draw your tongue in gently. Close your mouth.

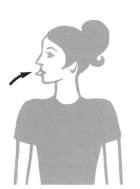

Step 3

Step 5
Exhale slowly and fully through the nose.

Repeat as often as you like.

WATCH OUT!

Cooling breath
- Those suffering high blood pressure should avoid this.
- Do not practise in very cold or hot air.

YOGIC BREATH

172

Bee breath (*Brahmari*)

Posture: seated with hands resting on knees (in *hasta mudra* if preferred – see p. 170).

Step 1
Close your eyes. Lips and mouth should be relaxed. Lips are gently closed and teeth remain slightly separated. Check that your jaw is relaxed.

Step 2
Inhale slowly and deeply through the nostrils.

Step 3
As you breathe out slowly, make a humming sound like a bee. The sound should last for as long as the out-breath and be smooth and even.

Step 4
Inhale slowly and deeply.

Step 5
Exhale making the sound of the bee and focusing your mind on this sound.

You can practise the bee breath for as long as you like.

WATCH OUT!

Bee breath
- Do not practise while lying down.
- Do not practise if you are suffering from an ear infection.

BENEFITS
- Helps insomnia.
- Calms the mind and soothes the spirit.
- Relaxes the body.
- Reduces blood pressure.

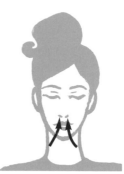

Step 2

want to know more?

Take it to the next level...

Go to...
▶ **Asana breathing** – page 30
▶ **The relaxation session** – page 158
▶ **The eight-fold path** – page 184

Other sources
▶ **Qualified yoga teacher**
   for specific breathing techniques
▶ **Videos/DVDs**
   for breathing exercises
▶ **Magazines**
   for specialist articles
▶ **Internet**
   for further information on chakras
▶ **Publications**
   visit www.thorsons.com for books on yoga

yoga at

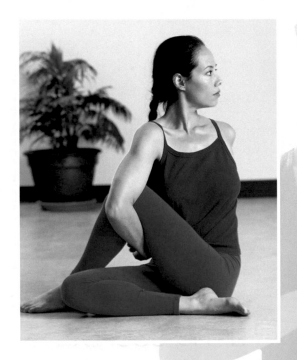

home

It is important to make yoga part of your daily routine so that if you happen to miss a session, you feel its absence and are keen to resume as soon as possible. One way of achieving this is to combine weekly classes with practice at home, using books and videos for reference if needed. This chapter is packed with advice on practising in your own home.

Home sessions

The key to success with yoga is perseverance in your practice. At home, it's better to set aside between 10 and 15 minutes a day rather than trying to manage hour-long bouts once a week or so.

Establishing a routine

Yoga practice is generally done in the morning or evening, whichever is more practical for you. If you have to get children ready for school in the morning, an evening session is probably your best option.

This does not mean setting aside an impossible amount of time. A series of short, personal practice sessions done daily is more realistic, and often more achievable, than sporadic sessions staged over a longer period.

WATCH OUT!

Relax
Remember the relaxation period at the end of a home session. If you spend 15 minutes on practice, leave three to five minutes for relaxation.

How long to practise

If you are a beginner, restrict your practice to 10 minutes at first. Gradually increase this to 15 or 20 minutes as your stamina and strength increase. If you have the opportunity, you could also try a longer session, perhaps up to an hour, once a week.

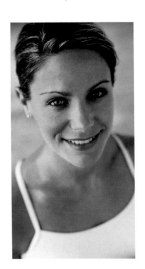

Where to practise

Set aside somewhere to practise. It should be airy, clean and free from disturbance such as noise or interruption from other people. For example, it would be impossible to practise with a TV on. Make sure your practice place is uncluttered. You could dedicate this area to yoga by placing a picture there that you particularly like. If this image is always present when you practise, it will focus your mind on the yoga and help concentration. In the early stages

◄ Your yoga session should leave you feeling invigorated and refreshed, not tired.

you might find it useful to practise the postures in front of a mirror so that you can check that you are doing them correctly.

What to wear

You should wear loose, comfortable clothing, with nothing on your feet. Try to keep what you wear just for your yoga practice; this will help focus your mind on what you are doing. White or cream-coloured clothing is ideal. Take off any jewellery that might distract you.

MUST KNOW

Useful items of home equipment
- A non-slip mat.
- A blanket (such as a plaid).
- A chair (to use for some more difficult postures).
- A small cushion (to support the head or buttocks).
- A belt.

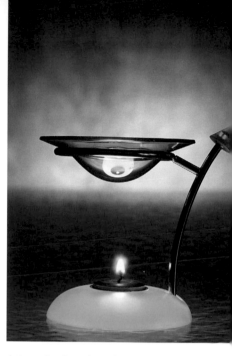

▲ Aromatic oils and candles are useful in creating an ambience at home that's conducive to concentrating and relaxing.

What to do before you start

Brush your teeth and clear your nasal passages. Empty your bladder and bowels. Remember, you should not have a heavy meal before your yoga session. You can eat a light snack an hour beforehand. It's also a good idea to let others in your house not to disturb you during your session Take the phone off the hook or put on the answering machine and switch off all mobiles.

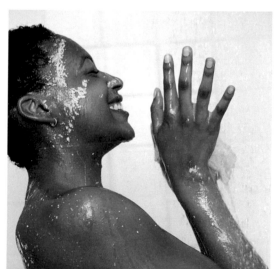

◀ If you have decided to practise early in the morning, a hot shower or bath will get rid of any overnight stiffness.

- Move slowly and mindfully. Don't rush from posture to posture – hold each one for a few seconds.
- Try to banish any outside thoughts; concentrate on the moment and what your body is doing – even the parts that aren't moving.
- Go as far as feels comfortable. Remember, pain is nature's way of saying that you are going too far and the people who demonstrate postures in books are generally experts with many years' experience. Do not try to compete with them.
- Breathe deeply and regularly; don't hold your breath.
- Use the in-breath (inhalation) for lifting and opening into a posture and the out-breath (exhalation) to fold and relax into it.

Which postures to do

Yoga is all about finding the correct balance and this balance should be reflected in the postures you choose. Listed below is a collection of asanas that would be ideal for a suggested home practice programme.

You should begin a session with a few limbering up exercises, especially if your session is in the morning. These could include Cat (p. 36), Butterfly (p. 40) and the Pelvic Lift (p. 38). Alternatively, you could do two or three rounds of Salutation to the Sun (p. 43).

SUGGESTED PRACTICE PROGRAMME

- A pose that centres you: Mountain (p. 48) or Tree (p. 50).
- A side stretch: Triangle (p. 56).
- A forward bend: Standing Forward Bend (p. 69) or Seated Forward Bend (p. 91).
- A backbend: Cobra (p. 122) or Upward-Facing Dog (p. 125).
- An inverted pose: Downward-Facing Dog (p. 144) or Plough (p. 147).
- A twist: such as Simple Twist (p. 128).
- Relaxation: in Corpse (p. 102) for at least three or four minutes.

When not to practise

If you have a medical condition, consult your doctor before taking up yoga. You should also take advice from a qualified yoga teacher as to what postures you should avoid or modify. For example, women who are menstruating should avoid inverted postures in the first few days. According to B. K. S. Iyengar, all the postures can be practised in the first three months of pregnancy. You will be able to judge for yourself whether a posture feels right for you. Cobbler, which strengthens pelvic muscles, is a good pose for pregnant women.

However, the joints become much looser during pregnancy in preparation for the birth so it is important that you do not overdo any postures because you find you are suddenly more flexible than usual.

Staying motivated

It is all too easy to start something with great enthusiasm, only to fall by the wayside after a few weeks. This is particularly true of self-improvement regimes which take some time to deliver the anticipated results.

▲ Pregnant women should seek the advice of a qualified yoga teacher on how to adapt the postures.

The secret to staying-power in yoga is discovering for yourself how much your life will benefit from it. Then, even if you later lapse for months or even years, one day you will find yourself coming back when the time is right or you find the right teacher.

MUST KNOW

Tips to help you stay motivated
● Find the right class for you and attend regularly. Make sure you leave work in plenty of time for an evening class and that you don't eat a big meal beforehand to give you an excuse not to attend.
● Make friends with others in your class.
● Try to attend a special day of yoga (often advertized in local yoga journals). A whole day spent devoted to yoga can be fulfilling and rekindle enthusiasm.
● Try out new postures in your daily routine and find out what effect they have on you.
● Get a friend interested and either practise together at home or attend the same class.

want to know more?

Take it to the next level...

Go to,...
▶ **The relaxation session** – page 158
▶ **Outfits and equipment** – page 22
▶ **The asanas** – page 34 onwards

Other sources
▶ **Magazines**
   for advice on asanas
▶ **Retreats**
   for relaxation and meditation practice
▶ **Videos/DVDs**
   for home practice direction
▶ **Internet**
   for equipment supplies
▶ **Publications**
   visit www.thorsons.com for books on yoga

living

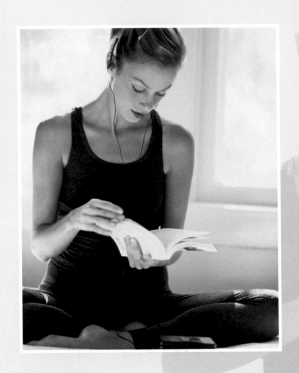

yoga

Yoga is not just a series of postures with odd names like cobra, locust and tree – it is a philosophy or way of life that is also very accessible. At its most basic level, it shows humans how to live to ensure a peaceful society and one that will protect the world's resources for future generations. This chapter explores some of the beliefs at the heart of yoga.

Yoga as a way of life

The key to yoga as a way of life can be found the meaning of the word itself. In Sanskrit, yoga translates as 'union' – the union between a human's individual consciousness and the Universal Consciousness. This can only happen by liberating oneself from a dependency on the trappings of modern life.

Yoga in everyday life

Yoga offers a means for people to control their senses and cultivate a detachment from life, allowing them the freedom to go beyond the confines of their own experience. Through yoga, people can free themselves from the human condition and all that this might entail: sadness, happiness, illness, poverty, wealth and so on.

The four stages

Yoga is a philosophy rooted very much in everyday life and according to the classical yoga tradition, there are four stages that a student must pass through:

Dharma: duty towards others and oneself; how you behave, and practise moderation in the way you live.

Artha: this stage is concerned with earning a living and being a householder – looking after yourself and family. This stage makes the student self-sufficient materially and teaches them love towards their family. It does not mean simply accumulating wealth but letting yourself be comfortable so you can enjoy life.

Kama: the enjoyment of life, best achieved with a healthy body and balanced mind. Yoga postures and breathing are important in achieving this.

Moksha: freedom from worldly pleasures. This can be achieved through controlling the senses and looking inward by practising meditation.

> **WATCH OUT!**
>
> **Keep it real**
> While yoga offers a technique for people to control their lives, this should not mean locking yourself away from reality. Yoga is meant to be an active part of all aspects of your life, not simply a compartment of it.

▼ *Kama* – pleasure or the fulfilment of desires – is a legitimate aim of life but only where it maintains or improves mental or physical wellbeing.

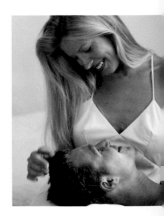

Types of yoga

As explained in the first chapter, in the West 'yoga' usually means hatha yoga. However, there are many different types, all leading to the same goal.

Traditionally. all these practices have been classified into four distinct paths.

Jnana yoga

The path of knowledge or wisdom. Jnana yoga is closely associated with the Vedanta philosophy of Hinduism and is regarded as the most direct way of reaching the goal of self-realization. At its core is meditation and self study aimed at revealing your real self from all that is unreal or illusory.

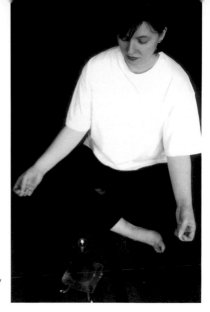

▲ The path of Jnana yoga calls for detachment and a heightened self-awareness.

Bhakti yoga

The path of devotion and worship of the divine. In the Hindu religion, there are thousands of gods and devotion to one or more of these is a way to yoga. This path is open to everyone – rich or poor, uneducated and educated. All that is required is faith and love.

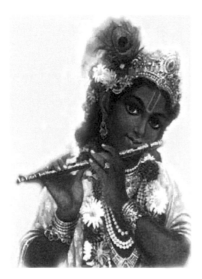

▲ Devotion to the Hindu deity, Krishna, is a main focus of Bhakti yoga.

Karma yoga

The path of action achieved through selfless service to others. The main thrust of Karma yoga is that a person's activities are undertaken for the greater good, without concern for personal benefit or reward. It is a suitable orientation for those with an active, outgoing nature.

Raja yoga

The yoga of mind and senses: the classical yoga. Hatha yoga is a branch of this. Although yoga does not involve elaborate rituals, Raja yoga consists of an eight-fold path, or the eight limbs of yoga.

The eight-fold path

In the West many associate yoga purely with the physical aspect – the postures known as asanas. In fact, this is just one of the eight limbs. Imagine this eight-fold path as a very wide path to begin with which everyone can travel down. It gets progressively narrower with fewer and fewer people reaching the end.

THE EIGHT-FOLD PATH

1. *Yamas*: rules aimed at destroying our lower nature.
2. *Niyamas*: rules or disciplines aimed at improving our individual nature.
3. *Asanas*: postures aimed at controlling the body. Most Westerners think yoga is just the asanas and so are confused over what yoga is. By practising the asanas or postures one learns control over the body.
4. *Pranayama*: breath control; teaches one how to control the breath and direct prana, or life energy.
5. *Pratyahara*: withdrawal of the senses.
6. *Dharana*: concentration.
7. *Dhyana*: meditation.
8. *Samadhi*: union with the Universal Consciousness or God. (Some beliefs refer to this Universal Consciousness as God.)

Yamas and niyamas

The first two limbs apply to everyone and consist of two sets of rules.

The first are the *yamas* – rules people must follow if they are to live in a peaceful society. They ensure that no harm comes to any living creature either through thought, word or deed.

The other set is the five *niyamas*, concerned with improving the individual's own character. Once the individual incorporates these rules into his or her daily life, then they are ready to progress along to the next stage of the eight-fold path.

Asanas, pranayama and pratyahara

The next three limbs of the path are *asanas, pranayama* and *pratyahara*. This withdrawal of the senses is where the student learns to

YAMAS

- Non-violence.
- Truthfulness.
- Non-stealing.
- Continence or chastity.
- Non-greed.

NIYAMAS

- Cleanliness (both of body and mind).
- Contentment.
- Austerity.
- Self-study.
- Devotion to God or the Ultimate Truth.

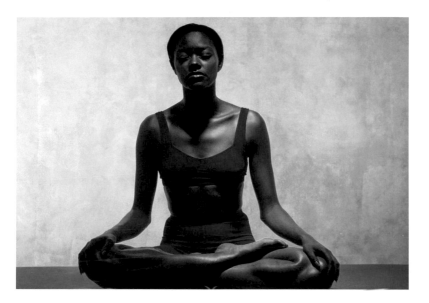

▲ Many yoga practitioners do not progress along the eight-fold path further than asanas, pranayama and pratyahara.

distance him- or herself from external life and the distractions of the body and senses. Now the student will continue the quest for the ultimate truth by turning inwards.

Dharana, dhyana and samadhi

The next two limbs of the eight-fold path are *dharana* (deep concentration) and *dhyana* (meditation). Once the follower has achieved this they may arrive at the final and eighth limb, *samadhi* or enlightenment where they are at one with the Universal Consciousness.

It is not an easy path to follow: the individual must rise above the passions of everyday life (and actively want to do this) in order to get there. Ultimately there has to be complete understanding of his or her own nature.

This in turn leads to the complete understanding of the Absolute or Universal truth of which we are all a part.

want to know more?

Take it to the next level...

Go to...
▶ **Types of yoga** – page 21
▶ **Yogic breathing exercises** – page 166
▶ **The asanas** – page 34 onwards

Other sources
▶ **Library or bookshop**
 for detailed studies of the belief system behind the different yoga systems
▶ **Magazines**
 for specialist articles and retreats to take your understanding to a higher level
▶ **Internet**
 for detailed information on yoga types
▶ **Publications**
 visit www.thorsons.com for books on yoga

Glossary of English-Sanskrit asana names

As explained in Chapter 3, yoga postures are known as asanas (pronounced a-sanas) and their names are often given in their native Sanskrit language. To the Westerner, such names may seem daunting at first but with a little practice, it won't take you long to remember them.

English-Sanskrit

Boat: Ardha navasana

Boat with oars: Paripurna navasana

Bow: Dhanurasana

Bridge: Setu bandha

Cat: Kummerasana

Cobbler: Baddha konasana

Cobra: Bhujangasana

Corpse: Savasana

Cow face: Gomukhasana

Downward-facing dog: Adho mukha svanasana

Easy pose: Sukhasana

Fish: Matsyasana

Flank stretch: Parsvakonasana

Half moon: Ardha chandrasana

Hero: Virasana

Legs up wall: Viparita karani

Locust: Salabhasana

Lying down hand–big toe: Supta padangusthasana

Lying twist: Jathara parivatanasana

Mountain: Tadasana

Plank: Chaturanga dandasana

Plough: Halasana

Pose of a child: Balasana

Rod: Dandasana

Salutation to the sun: Surya namaskar

Seated forward bend: Paschimottanasana

Seated spinal twist: Maricyasana

Seated wide–leg forward bend: Upavista konasana

Sideways forward bend: Parsvottanasana

Sideways hand–big toe: Anantasana

Simple twist: Bharadvajasana

Staff: Dandasana

Standing forward bend: Uttanasana

Swan: Hamsasana

Tree: Vrksasana

Triangle: Trikonasana

Upward-facing dog: Urdhva mukha svanasana

Warrior I: Virabhadrasana I

Warrior II: Virabhadrasana II

Wide-leg forward bend: Prasarita padottanasana

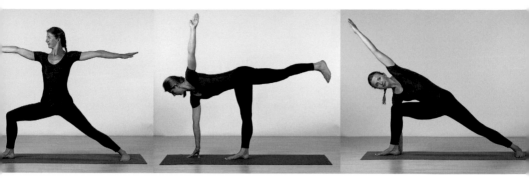

Sanskrit-English

Adho mukha savanasana:
Downward-facing dog

Anantasana: Sideways hand–big toe

Ardha chandrasana: Half moon

Ardha navasana: Boat

Baddha konasana: Cobbler

Balasana: Pose of a child

Bharadvajasana: Simple twist

Bhujangasana: Cobra

Chaturanga dandasana: Plank

Dandasana: Staff or Rod

Dhanurasana: Bow

Gomukhasana: Cow face

Halasana: Plough

Hamsasana: Swan

Jathara parivatanasana: Lying
twist

Kummerasana: Cat

Maricyasana: Seated spinal twist

Matsyasana: Fish

Paripurna navasana: Boat with
oars

Parsvakonasana: Flank stretch

Parsvottanasana: Sideways
forward bend

Paschimottanasana: Seated
forward bend

Prasarita padottanasana: Wide-
leg forward bend

Salabhasana: Locust

Savasana: Corpse

Setu bandha: Bridge

Sukhasana: Easy pose

Supta padangusthasana: Lying
down hand–big toe

Surya namaskar: Salutation to the
sun

Tadasana: Mountain

Trikonasana: Triangle

Upavista konasana: Seated wide-
leg forward bend

Urdhva mukha svanasana:
Upward-facing dog

Uttanasana: Standing forward
bend

Viparita karani: Legs up wall

Virabhadrasana I: Warrior I

Virabhadrasana II: Warrior II

Virasana: Hero

Vrksasana: Tree

Need to know more?

If you want to discover more about yoga, there is a wide range of resources available, especially if you have internet access. The following are particularly recommended.

Useful addresses

British Wheel of Yoga, 25 Jermyn Street, Sleaford, Lincolnshire NG34 7RU; tel: 01529 306851; email: office@bwy.org.uk
www.bwy.org.uk

International Kundalini Yoga Teachers' Association, Route 2, Box 4 Shady Lane, Espanola, NM 87532, USA; tel: (001) 505 753 0423; email: ikyta@3HO.org
www.kundaliniyoga.com

Iyengar Yoga Institute, 223a Randolph Avenue, London W9 1NL; tel: 020 7624 3080
www.iyi.org.uk

Sivananda Yoga Vedanta Centre, 51 Felsham Road, London SW15 1AZ; tel: 020 8780 0160; email: london@sivananda.org
www.sivananda.org

Viniyoga Britain, 105 Gales Drive, Three Bridges, Crawley RH10 1QD; tel: 01293 536664
www.viniyoga.co.uk

Yoga Plus, 177 Ditchling Road, Brighton BN1 6JB; tel: 01273 276175; email: yogaplus@pavilion.co.uk
www.yogaplus.co.uk

Magazines

Yoga & Health
Europe's leading yoga magazine featuring all aspects of yoga practice, very accessible introductions to subjects such as meditation plus articles on related topics.
www.yogaandhealthmag.org

Yoga International
A US yoga magazine featuring articles about yoga science, philosophy and Ayurveda.
www.yimag.org

Yoga Journal
The leading US yoga magazine which combines the essence of classical yoga with the latest understanding of modern science.
www.yogajournal.com

Yoga Magazine
The UK's newest monthly with innovative and entertaining articles, travel, health and beauty features, plus product reviews.
www.yogamagazine.co.uk

Equipment

Bodykind
Supplier of clothing, props and videos/DVDs for a range of mind-body practices including yoga.
www.bodykind.com

Simply Yoga
A specialist supplier of yoga props, clothing and videos/DVDs.
www.simply-yoga.co.uk

Yoga-Mad
Good source for yoga mats, books, videos and Iyengar yoga props.
www.yogamad.com

Exhibitions & events
Mind, Body & Soul Exhibitions
Useful website listing forthcoming MBS exhibitions in the UK.
www.mbsevents.co.uk
The Yoga Show
The official website of a major new annual show starting in 2004 devoted to yoga in the UK.
www.theyogashow.co.uk

Internet resources
www.ashtanga.com
An excellent site explaining all aspects of this style of yoga including listings of official teachers across the globe.
www.bksiyengar.com
The official site for Iyengar yoga, covering all aspects of this style.
www.bwy.org.uk
The British Wheel of Yoga is the governing body for yoga in the UK. This useful site provides listings of approved teachers and classes.
indigo.ie/~cmouze
Details of yoga courses and classes in Ireland.
www.viniyoga.co.uk
Useful site that explains this style of yoga in detail.
www.yogadirectory.com
Yoga search engine directory and website for the world-wide yoga community.

www.yogafinder.com
A resource to find yoga teachers worldwide.
www.yogascotland.org.uk
The website of the Scottish Yoga Teachers' Association with a database of classes, teachers and events in Scotland.
www.yogauk.com
YogaUK online magazine listing teachers, events, yoga holidays and yoga-related shopping.

Further reading
Currie, Barbara *10-Minute Yoga Workouts* (Thorsons)
Datta, Siri *Open Your Heart With Kundalini Yoga* (Thorsons)
Desikachar, T. K. V. *The Heart of Yoga* (Inner Traditions)
Devereux, Godfrey *Dynamic Yoga* (Thorsons)
Fraser, Tara *The Easy Yoga Work Book* (Duncan Baird Publishers)
Howe, Celia *Yoga for Slimmers* (Kyle Cathie)
Iyengar, B. K. S. *Light on Yoga* (Thorsons)
Judith, Anodea *Wheels of Life* (Llewellyn)
Kent, Howard *Illustrated Guide to Yoga* (Thorsons)
Mehta, Mira *Health Through Yoga* (Thorsons)
Sivananda Yoga Center *Yoga Mind & Body* (Dorling Kindersley)
Swenson, David *Ashtanga Yoga* (Ashtanga Yoga Productions)
Weller, Stella *Complete Yoga* (Thorsons)

Index

INDEX

191

☼ Collins need to know?

Want to know about other popular subjects and activities?
Look out for further titles in Collins' practical and accessible
Need to Know? series.

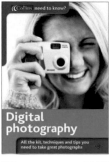

Digital photography
All the kit, techniques and tips you need to take great photographs

192pp £8.99
PB 0 00 718031 4

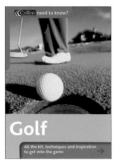

Golf
All the kit, techniques and inspiration to get into the game

192pp £8.99
PB 0 00 718037 3

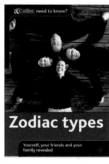

Zodiac types
Yourself, your friends and your family revealed

192pp £7.99
PB 0 00 718038 1

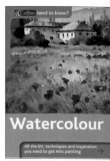

Watercolour
All the kit, techniques and inspiration you need to get into painting

192pp £8.99
PB 0 00 718032 2

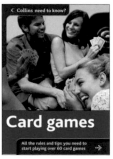

Card games
All the rules and tips you need to start playing over 60 card games

192pp £6.99
PB 0 00 719080 8

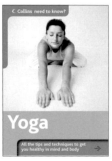

Yoga
All the tips and techniques to get you healthy in mind and body

192pp £8.99
PB 0 00 719091 3

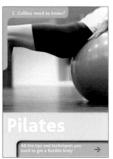

Pilates
All the tips and techniques you need to get a flexible body

192pp £8.99
PB 0 00 719063 8

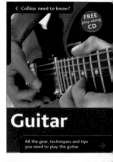

FREE play-along CD

Guitar
All the gear, techniques and tips you need to play the guitar

192pp £8.99
PB 0 00 719088 3

Forthcoming titles:

Birdwatching
DIY
Drawing & Sketching
Stargazing
Weddings
French
Italian

Spanish
Kama Sutra
Dog Training
Knots
World Atlas
World Factfile

To order any of these titles, please telephone **0870 787 1732**. For further information about all Collins books, visit our website: **www.collins.co.uk**